# Overcome Your

D1458655

**Professor Robert Bor**, DPhil, CPsychol, CSci, FBPsS, UKCP Reg, FRAeS, EuroPsy, is an internationally renowned clinical psychologist with expertise in the specialist area of aviation clinical psychology. Drawing on his e⟶ ⟶rience as a practising psychologist and a qualified pilot, he and his ⟶ agues provide an assessment and treatment service for helping r⟶ o overcome their fear of flying. They have developed innovative ⟶ ic methods based on modern psychological approaches. Robert ⟶ ⟶ellent clinical and research links with the Royal Free Hospital ⟶ alth Clinic, and the Fleet Street Clinic in London. He also has ⟶ in passenger and crew behaviour and is a consultant to British ⟶ ⟶, ⟶. He consults to several leading airlines and to international civil ⟶ation authorities. He teaches on the MSc in Air Transport Management ⟶ City University as well as on the MSc in Travel Health and Medicine at the Royal Free and University College Medical School. He is also involved in the selection of airline pilots, helping airlines develop mental health policies and training crew to deal with fearful passengers in managing 'air rage'. He has published more than 25 books and 150 academic papers in peer review journals.

**Dr Carina Eriksen** MSc, PsyD, CPsychol, is a Chartered Counselling Psycho⟶gist with many years' experience of the cabin crew profession. She holds ⟶ BSc in Psychology, a Master's degree in Psychology from London Metro⟶ tan University and a doctorate in Counselling Psychology. Carina work⟶ ⟶he NHS as well as in private practice. She provides therapy to adul⟶ ⟶dolescents, children and families, drawing on her speciality within cog⟶ ⟶e behavioural therapy and systemic orientations. She also offers ps⟶ ⟶gical support within organizational settings, including stress man-ag⟶ ⟶ and work-life conflict. She is a visiting lecturer on the MSc in Air Tr⟶ ⟶ Management at City University. Her work has been published in ⟶ and scientific journals. She is a chartered member of the British ⟶ical Society.

⟶ ⟶ **Oakes**, MA (Cantab), MSc, is a pilot with extensive experience f⟶ ⟶ a UK scheduled airline. She currently operates the Airbus A320 ⟶ aircraft on short haul and medium haul routes in Europe, Africa and ⟶ ⟶efore joining an airline, she spent several years as a flying instructor teaching technical subjects at an advanced level as well as practical flying skills to commercial pilots, one of fewer than 100 instructors qualified to do this in the UK. After completing a Master's degree project on the psychological perspectives of fear of flying, Margaret became a research student i⟶ ⟶, London. Her

H46 317 678 8

current research is focused on developing new and effective psychological approaches to treating fear of flying. She also teaches part of the Aviation Psychology modules in the MSc in Air Transport Management programme at City University.

# Overcoming Common Problems Series

*Selected titles*

A full list of titles is available from Sheldon Press,
36 Causton Street, London SW1P 4ST and on our website at
www.sheldonpress.co.uk

**The Assertiveness Handbook**
Mary Hartley

**Assertiveness: Step by step**
Dr Windy Dryden and Daniel Constantinou

**Backache: What you need to know**
Dr David Delvin

**Body Language: What you need to know**
David Cohen

**Calm Down**
Paul Hauck

**The Cancer Survivor's Handbook**
Dr Terry Priestman

**The Candida Diet Book**
Karen Brody

**Cataract: What you need to know**
Mark Watts

**The Chronic Fatigue Healing Diet**
Christine Craggs-Hinton

**The Chronic Pain Diet Book**
Neville Shone

**Cider Vinegar**
Margaret Hills

**The Complete Carer's Guide**
Bridget McCall

**The Confidence Book**
Gordon Lamont

**Confidence Works**
Gladeana McMahon

**Coping Successfully with Pain**
Neville Shone

**Coping Successfully with Panic Attacks**
Shirley Trickett

**Coping Successfully with Psoriasis**
Christine Craggs-Hinton

**Coping Successfully with Ulcerative Colitis**
Peter Cartwright

**Coping Successfully with Varicose Veins**
Christine Craggs-Hinton

**Coping Successfully with Your Hiatus Hernia**
Dr Tom Smith

**Coping Successfully with Your Irritable Bowel**
Rosemary Nicol

**Coping with Age-related Memory Loss**
Dr Tom Smith

**Coping with Birth Trauma and Postnatal Depression**
Lucy Jolin

**Coping with Bowel Cancer**
Dr Tom Smith

**Coping with Candida**
Shirley Trickett

**Coping with Chemotherapy**
Dr Terry Priestman

**Coping with Childhood Allergies**
Jill Eckersley

**Coping with Chronic Fatigue**
Trudie Chalder

**Coping with Coeliac Disease**
Karen Brody

**Coping with Compulsive Eating**
Ruth Searle

**Coping with Diabetes in Childhood and Adolescence**
Dr Philippa Kaye

**Coping with Diverticulitis**
Peter Cartwright

**Coping with Down's Syndrome**
Fiona Marshall

**Coping with Dyspraxia**
Jill Eckersley

**Coping with Eating Disorders and Body Image**
Christine Craggs-Hinton

**Coping with Epilepsy in Children and Young People**
Susan Elliot-Wright

**Coping with Family Stress**
Dr Peter Cheevers

**Coping with Gout**
Christine Craggs-Hinton

**Coping with Hay Fever**
Christine Craggs-Hinton

# Overcoming Common Problems Series

# Overcoming Common Problems Series

Overcoming Common Problems

# Overcome Your Fear of Flying

PROFESSOR ROBERT BOR, DR CARINA ERIKSEN
AND MARGARET OAKES

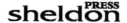

First published in Great Britain in 2009
Sheldon Press
36 Causton Street
London SW1P 4ST

*British Library Cataloguing-in-Publication Data*
A catalogue record for this book is available from the British Library

ISBN 978–1–84709–082–9

1 3 5 7 9 10 8 6 4 2

Typeset by Fakenham Photosetting Ltd, Fakenham, Norfolk
Printed in Great Britain by Ashford Colour Press

Produced on paper from sustainable forests

# Contents

*This book is dedicated to the many people who have shared with us their experiences of being afraid to fly. Working with them has given us an insight to the varied and individual ways in which being anxious or fearful about flying have an impact on thoughts, behaviour and emotions. This depth of understanding is the foundation of this self-help book, which we hope will help many others to overcome their fear.*

# 1

# Why another book about fear of flying?

Numerous books have been published on coping with a fear of flying, so why have we written another one? There are several reasons, and this chapter will outline how this book and our approach are different from others. No one has ever assessed how helpful the existing books are. Our experience with people who have a fear of flying shows that although some books provide useful information about flight safety, they do not explain the full range of psychological techniques which are known to help overcome fear and anxiety. Helping you to master these techniques is the main focus of this book; its purpose is to help you select and practise the techniques most likely to help you overcome your fear of flying. We also outline the way in which fear of flying can become a problem in the first place and how different people are affected.

Fear of flying is a surprisingly common problem, one that affects approximately 10 to 30 per cent of the adult population. For some, flying is unpleasant but manageable, while for others it is an incapacitating fear which they can neither face nor overcome. There may be serious and potentially disastrous social, financial and professional consequences for anxious or fearful flyers, while those who are truly phobic may avoid flying altogether. A fear of flying can spoil holidays, damage careers and put relationships under stress. The good news is that there are effective skills and techniques that you can use to reduce the fear and anxiety commonly associated with flying, all of which are described in this book.

A fear of flying is one of the most treatable psychological problems. For this reason almost everyone should be able to overcome their fear, provided that it has been properly assessed and treated using modern psychological methods. This book brings together the latest, proven methods for overcoming a fear of flying.

## What makes this book different?

This book takes an approach to the challenge of overcoming your fear of flying which you are unlikely to read in almost any other book on the topic. There are five main ways in which it is different:

1 It is written by a highly experienced and uniquely qualified team of experts, including pilots, crew and, of course, psychologists. We are committed to helping people overcome their fear of flying and apply tried and tested methods to achieve this. Each of us is qualified and experienced in more than one area, providing the broadest possible basis on which to offer you the skills and perspectives which can best help you. Together, we have more than 50 years of experience. We have published our research findings on treating fear of flying in many specialist medical and psychological journals as well as in books, and are often invited to talk about our work at conferences around the world.

2 We approach treatment of the problem differently from many others who deal with fearful flyers, and this book reflects that perspective. It will not baffle you with statistics about flight safety. We will certainly not 'argue' with any fears that you may have, and which may seem illogical or irrational to others (and sometimes to you too!). This book facilitates a tailored approach to self-help, built on a solid foundation of clinical practice and research. The aim is to motivate and empower you to confront and overcome the different elements that characterize your fear of flying.

3 We approach your fear of flying as a unique and specific problem that may be very different from other people's experience. You will see from some of the many examples that we quote in this book that a fear of flying affects people in many different ways; we tailor the solutions to your problem to your unique situation. We are not exponents of a 'one-size-fits-all' approach to treating a fear of flying. Before introducing ideas and skills for overcoming a fear of flying when we work with people professionally, we first listen very carefully to their experiences and stories about their difficulty. Of course, it is impossible to 'listen' to your personal story in a book. However, we reflect in this book the diverse contexts and struggles that we encounter with our clients, in order to convey the complex nature of the problem and allow you to begin to understand and overcome your own fear of flying.

4 The primary focus of the book is on psychological skills and techniques that you can apply to overcoming your fear of flying. These skills are derived from the findings of modern psychological

research. They focus on what you can *do* and how you can *think* about situations differently so as to help you on your way. You will be able to see and measure your progress along the way. You may be relieved to know that this process will not start with questions about your childhood, even though there may be some vague relevance to your earlier years. Modern psychological approaches focus on what is happening to you now and what you can do to bring about change, rather than on developing deep insight into your problems. You may find that some of the ideas you come across in the book can even be used and applied to help you in other areas of your life which present a challenge for you.

5 This is an extensive and practical self-help book derived from modern evidence-based clinical practice. It is designed to help you (the anxious flyer), or a person who accompanies an anxious flyer, to gain confidence in the proven skills and techniques needed to overcome your fear. The book will engage you in reflection and encourage you to try out a few skills and tasks. It will help you to develop an understanding of your own way of thinking about flying and enable you to select and try out the psychological techniques that are most likely to help you. At various points in each chapter, you will find 'Stop and Think' exercises designed to help you apply the information and techniques to your own situation.

There are many treatment programmes available for fearful flyers which aim to reduce anxiety about flying, and they do work for many people. Most of these take the form of a one-day course for groups which covers in the limited time available the information and techniques that most people find useful. A typical course will start with lectures on flight safety and how aircraft fly, move on to some relaxation training and finish with a short flight taken in a specially chartered aeroplane with just the anxious flyers and course staff. These courses are effective for many people and are probably the most accessible treatment for fear of flying. A course like this may be a useful further step for you to take in overcoming your fear of flying.

However, we frequently meet people who find that taking the step from flying on a fear of flying course to independent travel by air has been too big a challenge. In fact, research shows that although these courses are very successful, 10 to 40 per cent of people surveyed who complete them are not flying independently two years later. There may be a number of reasons for this:

- Without individual preparation it can be very difficult to identify the techniques which are most likely to work for your own fear of flying.
- You may be trying to use too many of the techniques taught on the course or not selecting those most appropriate for you.
- Some of the techniques most likely to work for you may not have been included in the course.
- For some people, there may be too much information in the course lectures, which can itself sometimes increase anxiety.

A proportion of the people we work with tell us that flying in a supportive group with trained and sympathetic staff is not enough practice at flying to allow them to confidently fly independently.

If you think a fear of flying course might help you, working with this book or with a psychologist, who can carry out an accurate assessment of your fear of flying, will help you prepare for it. You will be able to build an understanding of your own fear and to identify the techniques which are most likely to work for you so that you can concentrate on practising those on your course. This is one reason why we carry out individual assessments before people come to our fear of flying courses. You can also use this book to help you practise what you have learnt between your course and your next flight and to prepare for future journeys. This book will help you to manage the additional challenges of flying independently and assist you to identify any additional help you may need to do this. Some people have found that additional sessions with a psychologist or taking a scheduled flight with a trained escort help to bridge the gap.

Because fear of flying varies so widely, no course can cover everything that everybody needs. We cannot cover everything in this book either. What we can do, though, is outline the psychological techniques that are most likely to work and show you how to use them. Once you have been introduced to these skills, you can try them out for yourself. You may also need to use other sources of information, such as those listed under 'Other sources of help' at the end of this book.

## What's in the rest of this book?

The rest of this book contains information, techniques to practise, and advice. Not all of it will be useful to everyone, but you will find guidance on how to select and try the techniques most likely to work for you. The book is entirely practical in its focus. It is oriented to helping you first to understand the source or causes of your fear of flying from a psychological perspective. Through case studies, it describes in detail the different presentations of the problem, helping you to recognize how your own difficulty with flying affects you. It then goes on to highlight the wide variety of potential triggers which must be identified and treated in order to overcome the problem. The final chapters cover the information, skills and techniques you will need to begin formulating your own individual treatment plan. Briefly, here's what each chapter contains:

- **Chapter 2** explores the experience of being anxious or fearful about flying. It contains a number of case studies which illustrate each individual's experience and how varied fear of flying can be. It also describes the impact fear of flying can have on many people's lives.
- **Chapter 3** helps you to understand what fear of flying is and looks at how large a proportion of the population are affected. It introduces the psychological techniques used to help people overcome a fear of flying, and encourages you to start to consider your own experience, as the first step towards understanding your own fear. This chapter finishes with a longer case study which tells the story of one fearful flyer. We have included this to show you how the techniques in this book can be used to overcome a fear of flying; reading it will help you start to identify the skills and techniques which are most likely to work for you.
- **Chapter 4** explores fear of flying from a psychological perspective, without using technical language. It aims to help you understand your own fear and asks you to continue to consider your own experience, so that in later chapters you can start working on your own problem.
- **Chapters 5 and 6** take this further by discussing what causes fear of flying and what might be happening to reinforce your anxiety and prevent you from overcoming it. Chapter 5 looks at the thoughts, behaviour and bodily sensations experienced by people who are anxious about flying. Chapter 6 describes the thoughts and behaviours that may reinforce your anxiety. Use these chapters to explore your own fear of flying in more detail. Although they might not seem to be 'teaching' you very much, they will help you to understand your own thoughts, behaviours and sensations. This knowledge will help you select the skills and techniques you need from the chapters that follow.
- **Chapters 7 and 8** will 'teach' you the skills and techniques required to overcome your fear of flying. Chapter 7 gives you practical advice on challenging and managing anxious thoughts and

tackling unhelpful behaviour. Chapter 8 describes several techniques to reduce physical tension and the bodily signs of anxiety.

- **Chapter 9** answers the questions we have most often been asked about how aircraft fly, pilots, cabin crew and so on. It also answers the most common 'what happens if …?' questions and shows you how to construct your own answers to questions you may have.

- **Chapter 10** starts with another longer case study, describing how a fearful flyer used the techniques and information in this book to overcome his fear. This story will show you how the skills we describe can be brought together. The rest of this final chapter contains hints and tips to remind you how to apply the techniques in this book when you actually take a flight. It starts with planning your journey and reminds you how to deal with the build-up to your flight. It lists techniques to use before and during the flight and helps you to cope better within the airport environment. It has useful information for people travelling with anxious flyers, as well as advice for those who have worked through this book but then decide not to travel.

Good luck, and we hope that you enjoy working through the book. You have already committed yourself to trying to understand your fear and to work towards overcoming it. This motivation will add to the likely success of your hard work.

# 2

# What is it like having a fear of flying?

'Fear of flying' is a term used for many more specific fears; no two people are alike in this regard. People who have a fear of flying may have unique and specific causes of their difficulty, but they all share a problem that manifests itself in one way: they don't like the idea of travelling in an aircraft. They mostly differ, however, in the possible causes of their fear of flying; in the events or circumstances that trigger anxiety and worry; how they cope; and in those factors that prevent change or recovery from their fear. This chapter will help you to understand the different circumstances and unique situations that cause a fear of flying. It will highlight the unique and sensitive stories of some other fearful flyers.

While reading through this chapter and the case studies, you will become aware of the diverse nature of the problem and the impact that it has on people from many different backgrounds. The case studies are based on real experiences of people we have treated, but we have deliberately changed many of the personal details so as to preserve confidentiality.

## Fear of flying case studies

In the following case, Rachel's fear of flying had been long-standing. However, it became worse when her husband was transferred abroad to work. This led to her seeking treatment for the problem which she successfully overcame.

> Rachel, a 28-year-old housewife, had been afraid of flying for as long as she could remember. She couldn't explain why she was afraid to fly, but was convinced that flying was dangerous and frightening. Seeing an aircraft overhead would make her anxious and driving past the local airport was something she actively avoided, even though it was on the direct route to the supermarket where she did most of her shopping. When her husband's career required a move to Gibraltar, she refused to go with him as she felt unable to face the journey by air. Her husband's response was to arrange an earlier departure date, and he walked out

on Rachel and their three children. In an attempt to 'face up to her fears', Rachel persuaded a friend to drive her to the local airport – a busy regional airfield with frequent flights by small and medium jet aircraft. Before they could sit down inside the airport, Rachel had a panic attack and they left quickly. This experience led Rachel to seek treatment which focused on providing her with techniques to manage and reduce her fear and provided some information on flight safety. She found techniques focused on identifying and changing anxious thoughts particularly useful. She still uses these methods and is now able to fly with only mild anxiety. Rachel moved her family to Gibraltar very shortly after treatment.

Many people who have flown confidently for several years or even for all of their lives develop a fear of flying quite suddenly, and sometimes without an identifiable reason. A psychologist or therapist can help in pinpointing the likely cause or trigger, which can be both reassuring for the individual and also relevant to the course that therapy will take. In Jason's case, however, his fear developed after a flight that he took had to make an emergency landing.

Jason, a 47-year-old company director, had flown frequently and confidently for more than 20 years, with many business trips to long-haul destinations. Returning to the UK on one occasion, he was involved in an emergency landing and evacuated with the other passengers and crew using the emergency exits and slides. Jason became very apprehensive about his next trip, which was scheduled to take place only three weeks after this experience. At the thought of packing for this journey, Jason became 'tearful and shaky' and would vividly recall the traumatic ending to his last flight. He felt under great pressure from his fellow directors to travel on schedule, as the trip involved a meeting which required his technical expertise to complete negotiations on a major contract. He had mixed feelings about the contract as success would mean even more flights on business. Jason considered his response 'cowardly', especially as his colleagues took the attitude that he had survived the experience and it was unlikely to happen again. Once he was able to accept that his fear was a very rational response to a frightening experience, Jason began to feel 'less pressured' to fly. With techniques to manage his anxiety and deal with any tendency to recall his experience, Jason took a short 'practice' flight and subsequently felt confident enough to continue with his business trip as planned.

Less dramatic, but for some passengers no less terrifying, is the aircraft encountering turbulence in flight. This encounter can lead some passengers to become fearful and feel vulnerable. Some may worry that something bad will happen to the aircraft. Their imagination may even extend beyond this; for a few, their fear escalates into thinking that the plane might crash. Turbulence does not cause accidents, but the unpleasant physical sensation of the aircraft bumping through the air is one of the most common triggers of a fear of flying, as Annette discovered.

Annette, a 35-year-old schoolteacher, had been flying confidently for over ten years. She became fearful of flying after a holiday flight to Spain encountered unexpected turbulence. She witnessed one of the cabin attendants screaming in pain after he had been scalded by a stream of hot coffee from the pot he had been holding. When she arrived at her destination, Annette had to 'peel her hands away from the arm rests' which she had been holding. She spent her holiday worrying about the flight back and became a 'white knuckle flyer' from then on. Annette was determined to take her seven-year-old autistic son on holiday but wanted to 'sort herself out' first. She found that information on the causes of turbulence and how aircraft are designed to handle it reduced her anxiety. Relaxation techniques completed her return to the role of 'confident flyer'.

Choosing to fly (or choosing not to fly) at least leaves some people in control of their travels and therefore better able to control or avoid their fears associated with flying. However, the absence of choice can also be a significant factor in the development of a fear of flying. For example, having to travel for business or to attend an important family function can be stressful and generate significant anxiety. Careers and relationships may sometimes be at stake where a person suffers from a fear of flying. Suffering a panic attack in public can lead to feelings of shame and embarrassment that only make the fear more intense, as Linda experienced.

Linda, a 39-year-old manager, had recently developed a fear of flying despite having flown confidently since early childhood. She attributed her anxiety to a traumatic plane journey when returning from Geneva, where she had visited her boyfriend for the weekend. Shortly after take-off Linda fell asleep and she remembers feeling hot and sweaty when she awoke 30 minutes later. She stood up to go to the bathroom and fainted. She recalls being surrounded by cabin crew who were 'fussing' about her wellbeing. Although the crew were sympathetic and caring, Linda recalls feeling embarrassed and ashamed at having attracted 'unnecessary attention' to herself. When she got off the aircraft she vowed to never travel again and had not been on a plane for the past six months. This had put a strain on her relationship, as her boyfriend was unable to travel to London every weekend. The fainting had led Linda to believe she was 'losing control' and the consequent attention from the crew had made her worry about other people's (both crew and passengers') perception of herself (as 'an attention seeker', 'a mad woman'). As time passed, the avoidance of air travel gradually served to strengthen her beliefs. The absence of fainting and feelings of embarrassment and shame were wholly attributed to being on the ground, and therefore Linda was convinced that travelling by plane was a dangerous activity that would cause her to 'lose control again'. Once Linda was able to identify the underlying cause of her difficulty she managed to control her anxiety, which in turn allowed her to conquer the fear of flying.

Not every fearful flyer is afraid of being on an aircraft. Instead some may be averse to unique and specific aspects of air travel. This in turn may lead to a fear of flying because flying is obviously associated with air travel in general. The origins of the problem may be diverse and, for example, stem from a fear of being away from a loved one (perhaps because on a previous occasion this led to an illicit extra-marital liaison) or, in John's case, a bad experience with security staff at an airport.

John, a 50-year-old businessman, was finding it increasingly difficult to travel abroad as his work required. For the past 15 years John had frequently travelled to and from the United States for both meetings and leisure. Although he described himself as 'never having been a confident flyer', John explained how his fear had worsened over the past two years, often leading him to 'dread' business trips many days prior to travelling abroad. The anxiety caused sleeplessness, stress, and concentration difficulties. For John, the worst part of travelling was going through 'security'. He said he felt intimidated and scrutinized by the 'ruthless' demands placed on him: 'Remove your belt', 'Take off your shoes', 'No sir – you have to place your laptop and mobile phone in the plastic drawers', 'Step aside – we need to check you again'. By the time he got to the gate, John was dripping in sweat, exhausted, stressed and annoyed.

It appeared that the airport security procedure reminded John of experiences with his father during childhood. He recalls how his father used endless 'orders' to maintain authority at home, and that this used to make John feel 'powerless' and 'fearful'. The stress arising from feeling 'intimidated' and 'helpless' meant that John would often board the aircraft in an anxious and worried frame of mind. This heightened anxiety, along with John's general lack of confidence on board an aircraft, appeared to be the problem that underlay his fear of flying. Techniques for dealing with the security procedures, along with stress management, became an important tool for helping John to overcome his fear of flying.

Parents are often curious about whether children are born with a fear of flying or whether it is a problem that develops later on. There are different theories that account for how fears and phobias develop. It is generally agreed among psychologists, though, that children can experience a fear of flying. It may be that such children acquire this fear from a parent whom they observe closely, struggling with his or her own difficulty with flying, or perhaps the fear is passed on genetically. Whatever the explanation, a distressed child on board an aircraft is always a testing experience for all those affected. Of course, the distress may be triggered by a number of factors or situations, such as ear discomfort during take-off or descent, unfamiliar surroundings, separation from a favoured toy or comfort blanket, or being confined to one's seat. But a child who suffers from a fear of flying affects the whole family, as Jacob's story illustrates.

Jacob was only three years of age when he made clear to his parents that he hated being in an aeroplane. His parents had bought a private game farm in South Africa which had its own airstrip. He was clearly apprehensive when he boarded the overnight flight from London to Johannesburg together with his parents and older brother and sister. Exhibiting extreme fear of separation, he was tearful and restless, clutched at his comfort blanket and could not be prised apart from his mother, who had to carry him on to the aircraft. He screamed at take-off when he was required to sit on his own with his seat belt fastened.

Things got worse when the family arrived in Johannesburg and transferred to a small propeller-driven aircraft to take them to the game farm. He was again tearful and started to scream when they boarded, causing embarrassment to his older siblings and exasperation to his parents, who felt that they could not comfort him. The family sought psychological help for his problem with flying when they returned to the UK, as they realized that they would need to find strategies to help him to cope better with flying if they were to enjoy many more visits to the farm. A psychologist met his parents and helped them develop methods for distraction and relaxation to help Jacob to fly more easily. The session also revealed that his mother had many fears and phobias of her own and she was worried that she had 'infected' Jacob with her anxiety. Helping his mother to cope better with her own anxieties helped Jacob to manage his flights to the farm.

Some people go to great lengths to conceal from others their fear of flying. They may tell friends, family and employers elaborate stories about why they cannot fly. Ignoring the problem seldom results in any improvement, and so their motivation to overcome the problem may be prompted by external factors and pressure. Brad's case illustrates how mounting pressure and distress led him to seek specialist help for his fear of flying.

> Brad sought help for his fear of flying when he was in his twenties. He worked as a builder and felt ashamed when his fellow workers spoke enthusiastically about the holidays they were planning, or those from which they had returned. He avoided taking holidays abroad and would make excuses to his fellow workers, 'blaming' his girlfriend whom he claimed had a fear of flying. Things came to a head when he was invited to a stag weekend in Berlin with a group including several others with whom he worked. He looked into the possibility of taking a train to Berlin, but could not think of a good reason to tell the others why he would want to take a lengthy train journey on his own. Brad became agitated when his fellow workers enquired whether he had booked his flight. He started taking off days from work, claiming that he was sick. His situation became worse as he did not get paid for the days he was not at work, and his girlfriend suggested he see his GP to help him with his mood. His GP was sympathetic and helpful. He encouraged Brad to explain to his girlfriend what was wrong with him, so as to reduce the sense of shame he had about having a problem with flying. His GP also referred him to a psychologist who helped him to understand the cause of his fear and how best to overcome it.

Psychologists will often help their clients to distinguish between the symptoms of a problem and the underlying cause. In Steve's case, the underlying cause of his fear of flying was possibly the use of recreational drugs, which had left him vulnerable to anxiety and low mood. Many anxious travellers will 'self medicate' with alcohol, certain non-prescribed medications or even illicit drugs in order to lower their anxiety. Unfortunately, using these substances to overcome one's fear may not always be effective and in some cases may even make the symptoms of fear worse. Where this occurs, it is helpful to look at the solutions that fearful flyers have attempted to see whether their own remedy to their problem has unexpectedly made the problem even worse.

> Steve was the lead guitarist in a band and developed a fear of flying soon after his band was invited to do a gig in Dublin. He had travelled quite extensively until then, but became panicked and felt immobilized

by fear when it came to taking the band abroad. His previous flight was a long-haul trip to the Maldives, which he managed with his girlfriend. He felt that his fear was triggered when, on the return leg, a female pilot made an announcement to passengers. On realizing that the pilot was female, he said, 'I suddenly had this overwhelming fear; I know it's a bit sexist but I just didn't feel as safe. I prayed most of the way home and bargained with God that if we got home all right I wouldn't fly again.'

Other band members put him under pressure to arrange the gig. Steve started to feel torn between wanting to travel and not to let the band down, on the one hand, and a worry that his breaching his 'agreement' with God would result in catastrophe. He had four sessions with a therapist who helped him with his fear. She explained to him that the trigger event – his feeling more vulnerable with a female pilot – was not the cause of his fear but was more likely the first time that he recognized the anxiety which had been steadily but silently increasing over the previous months. Of special note was the fact that he had been using copious amounts of recreational drugs in the previous year, including ecstasy and cocaine. This had made him more vulnerable to anxiety and low mood, which had manifested in a fear of flying. Psychological treatment was effective in rapidly helping Steve's mood to improve and in enabling him to control his anxiety symptoms. He was able to travel to Dublin with his band.

Doctors can prescribe specific medications to help passengers to cope better with certain unpleasant symptoms that may be associated with a fear of flying. These include medications to help relieve blocked sinuses, which may create extreme discomfort in the ears; medications to help the person to sleep on board the aircraft; medications to overcome air sicknesses; and short- and long-term treatments for the symptoms of anxiety and panic attacks. In some cases, such treatments can help fearful flyers to feel less distressed and reduce the intensity of their fear of flying to manageable proportions. However, medication may not always be the best way to treat anxiety. For some people, the changes a doctor makes to your medication – whether or not it is prescribed for anxiety – can affect the symptoms of anxiety.

Saira was born in Pakistan and came to live in the UK soon after she was married. She never felt comfortable when travelling on aircraft and would not contemplate a journey without her husband or grown-up children. Her doctor would prescribe a sedative and sleeping pill whenever she had to travel. After she developed asthma and heart problems, her doctor was reluctant to continue to prescribe these medications to help her cope with her fear of flying. This posed a problem for Saira, as members of her extended family lived in many different countries.

She would become breathless, sweaty, agitated, develop motion sickness and sometimes become tearful before boarding an aircraft. She once had to leave the aircraft while it was still at the boarding gate as she felt claustrophobic; overwhelmed by her feelings, she had a panic attack. Realizing that she had to find another way to cope with her fear of flying, she enrolled on an airline's fearful flyers course and also saw a psychologist. While she continues to fly only if accompanied by at least one family member, she no longer avoids overseas trips and has not suffered another panic attack.

People who suffer from a fear of flying do not necessarily experience higher levels of anxiety and stress in other areas of their lives. Adebisi's story clearly illustrates this. In spite of the obvious risks associated with travelling to a relatively unstable country with all its attendant health and safety risks, she was determined to spend her gap year helping a community. However, travelling there by plane was an almost insurmountable challenge.

Adebisi finished school and was looking forward to her gap year, some of which was to be spent helping to build schools in Rwanda. She had no fear of living away from home for the first time, nor of the risks of living in a foreign and unknown country. However, the prospect of taking a flight on her own proved overwhelming. In the days leading up to her trip, she started to feel very anxious and thought about cancelling her trip. Her family and friends tried to reason with her using statistics about flight safety, pointing out that car journeys posed a much greater risk than flying. She accepted their explanations but was not reassured by logic and reasoning.

When the day came for her to travel, Adebisi was unable to board the aircraft. A flight attendant failed to persuade her to fly and so her baggage was removed from the hold of the aircraft and her parents collected her to take her home. Her anxiety vanished completely as soon as she left the airport, but later in the day she started to feel sad that she had let herself and others down. Realizing that she had developed a fear of flying, she searched the internet for information on flight safety, anxiety, phobias and fear of flying. While much of the information she came across was helpful to her and gave her some insight into her problem, she recognized that she needed to speak to someone outside her family who was professionally trained to deal with her problem. Six weeks later, she was able to fly to Rwanda.

Logical reasoning and an explanation as to how planes fly may not be enough to quell the nerves of some fearful flyers. In fact many people who have a fear of flying have a comprehensive understanding of flight safety, but simply do not believe that such logic and reassurance applies to them. This is one reason why some fearful flyers gain only limited relief by attending fear of flying workshops and airline training events. In some cases, a person's fear of flying may become 'infectious' and may undermine the confidence and coping strategies of his or her travelling companions.

> Wilbur was always sympathetic towards his wife's fear of flying and never put her under pressure to travel. Riva was convinced that she would perish in an air accident, as her father had while on a business trip in Japan many years ago. No amount of logic or reasoning was sufficient to persuade Riva to fly when she felt overwhelmed by her fears. She would still fly, but only very occasionally and never more than once a year. On one occasion, Wilbur became worried that he would be overwhelmed by his wife's anxieties on a trip. He feared that she would panic on board the aircraft and that he would be left on his own to help her if she suffered a panic attack. The couple realized that they both had a fear of flying, although for different reasons, and jointly participated in a one-day fear of flying course to help them with their problem.

A fear of flying can be considered a form of psychological problem, or at least a personal or lifestyle limitation. However, it need not all be bad news for the sufferer. Clinical experience has shown that when faced with a fear or phobia, some people experience unexpected benefits in other areas of their life. The psychological therapy and counselling that they undergo for their fear of flying, and the insights and confidence that they gain, can help them to move ahead in their relationships and career, as Idan's case demonstrates.

> Idan was promoted to regional account manager for a private bank, a role which required extensive travel. He had previously been comfortable taking holiday trips with his boyfriend, but business trips posed a problem. He felt worse every time he had to fly abroad. He felt anxious when he was away from home because he felt insecure in the relationship. Idan dreaded his secretary telling him when he would next be flying. He even thought about giving up his job so that he would not have to travel abroad as much.
>
> He eventually told his manager about his difficulties with overseas travel, and the manager offered to pay for some sessions with a psychologist. During these sessions, it emerged that Idan's anxiety stemmed from his parents' divorce, which made him fear for his own relationship. The psychologist offered to work with Idan and his boyfriend as

a couple to help establish whether the fears were founded and to help them to manage periods of physical separation. They developed ways to maintain emotional intimacy in their relationship while Idan was abroad. This helped him to focus on his work while he was away, building on previous success in his career, which in turn led to him being promoted to a role that entailed far less travel.

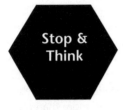

**Stop & Think**

Have you tried any treatments for fear of flying? Did they work? What aspect of your fear remains the strongest in your mind? What do want to achieve? Would you be prepared to practise techniques that might help so that you were proficient at them before flying?

This chapter has introduced you to the way in which people with a fear of flying will be very different from one another. It has also looked at the ways in which fear of flying can have negative effects on a person's personal and professional life. The next chapter explains what we mean by fear of flying, to begin helping you to understand your own anxiety and fear.

# 3

# Fear of flying and how this book can help you overcome it

Explaining what we mean by 'fear of flying' is a useful starting point for many fearful flyers we have worked with. It is often the first step towards understanding your own fear or anxiety about flying. It can also reduce the shame or embarrassment many people tell us is associated with being afraid to do something that others seem to do effortlessly. This chapter describes fear of flying and why overcoming and understanding it matters. It also asks you to start thinking about your goals in overcoming your fear and introduces the techniques which we will explain and illustrate in detail later in the book.

## What is fear of flying?

The term 'fear of flying' covers a vast range of reactions to travelling in an aircraft. It includes those who are slightly anxious about flying, those who avoid making unnecessary flights and those who will fly only when they must and are very anxious when doing so. It can even involve panic attacks at the thought of taking a flight, or a complete refusal to fly. People with a fear of flying share a dislike of travelling in an aircraft and find it makes them feel anxious or scared. Apart from having this in common, however, they will be very different in what caused their anxiety or fear and in the way they think about flying.

Most people who have a fear of flying describe their fear as 'irrational'. They recognize that the risk of harm associated with air travel is much less than the risks involved in daily activities, such as driving to and from work or the risk of contracting a disease. They may even feel ashamed about having a fear of flying, but equally they may be at a loss as to how to overcome or control it. It would be more logical to have a fear of driving to or from the airport or a fear of being struck by lightning while playing golf, where statistically the risk to life far exceeds that imagined by fearful flyers. However, knowing the statistics may not reduce anxiety or fear, because this knowledge on its own cannot always change the way a person thinks.

From a psychologist's perspective, fear of flying is a specific phobia of the situational type. That means it is fear that is triggered by a particular situation, in this case planning or taking (or attempting to take) a flight. To be formally identified as a phobia, a fear must be considered excessive in relation to the risk involved and be an ongoing problem for the person concerned. Most people who have a phobia will recognize that their fear is out of proportion to the actual danger and it will significantly interfere with their quality of life. Unfortunately, as you will discover in Chapters 4 and 5, simply recognizing that a fear may be 'irrational' will not necessarily help reduce fear and anxiety. It can actually make the situation worse by adding shame or embarrassment to the stress of dealing with a feared situation.

Fear of flying doesn't have to be so marked and distressing that it justifies a diagnosis of phobia to have a damaging effect on someone's life. Depending on the attitudes of those around you, even mild anxiety in relation to flying can create stress when planning holidays or business travel. People whose experiences don't completely match the clinical definition of fear of flying still find it unpleasant and anxiety-provoking, and will often avoid flying.

## Who is afraid to fly?

The simple answer is that just about anyone can become afraid to fly. Fear of flying has been studied and measured only in Western Europe, North America and Australia. Surveys have shown that approximately 2.5 per cent of the general population in these areas will have a specific phobia triggered by flying. Another 15 per cent will avoid flying to some extent and an additional 25 to 30 per cent may be anxious when flying. In the UK alone, that means that over 1.5 million people have an identifiable phobia of flying, over 9 million will avoid travelling by air to some degree and as many as 27 million people suffer from some degree of anxiety when faced with the prospect of taking a flight.

Surveys in Western Europe, North America and Australia show that women are almost twice as likely as men to be anxious or fearful about flying. The reason for this has not been completely determined. Women may be more likely to admit to anxiety about flying, possibly because it's more acceptable for women to fear flying than men. It may be because women are more likely to consider the consequences to their families of accidents or they may be more likely to associate flying with being stressed or unhappy. Perhaps a greater proportion of women agree to take part in surveys on this topic!

Outside Western Europe, North America and Australia, fear of flying has not been extensively measured. However, it is likely that in most areas of the world where major airlines operate, a similar proportion of the population is anxious or afraid of air travel.

In summary, fear of flying is very common. People from all backgrounds can become anxious about flying and if you talk about it, you're likely to find that a large proportion of your friends and family are anxious about air travel, even if only slightly. As you will see later in this book, there are many things you can do to reduce the anxiety associated with flying.

## Why does fear of flying matter?

Fear of flying matters because it stops people being able to travel on aircraft. It is important because it has an impact on people's quality of life. The case studies in the previous chapter illustrate just some of the ways in which fear of flying can have damaging effects on people's lives. It can spoil holidays, put relationships under stress and even damage careers. Disagreements over where to go on holiday can happen because one person wants to avoid flying. Once a holiday has been planned, someone who is anxious about the flight will probably find that he or she gets more anxious as the time to depart approaches. This often means that you can't look forward to taking a holiday at all, which can interfere with 'normal life'. Then you have to get through the flight itself and even when you get there, you still have to worry about flying home. Many people tell us that the last part of their holiday is usually spoilt because they become more and more anxious about the return flight.

Not wanting to fly to go on holiday is only one way in which fear of flying can put relationships with friends and family under stress. It can make keeping in touch difficult and even stop people going to important family events such as weddings and funerals. As Rachel and Brad describe in Chapter 2, being anxious about flying can severely damage relationships with family, colleagues and friends.

Professional relationships and careers can also suffer when someone is afraid to fly. As Jason describes in Chapter 2, colleagues can be unsympathetic and there can be a lot of pressure to travel in order to win contracts or fix problems. People tell us that this can quite suddenly become a problem when their professional role demands travel with little or no notice, perhaps when companies merge or new contracts involve international customers. We have also heard people say that they have avoided a promotion because the new role would involve flying, or that they would promote a very good individual but are unable to do so because that person will not fly.

## What's it like to fly with reduced anxiety?

You may already know the answer to this. Many people who have become anxious about flying tell us that they used to be able to fly confidently. This can often mean that they become very self-critical, thinking that they should still be able to fly without anxiety.

The fact is that flying involves stress or anxiety for most people, whether they are rushing to the airport, wondering if they've chosen the right holiday, being separated from loved ones, worrying about a business meeting or being a fearful flyer. If you are aiming to be able to fly with no fear or anxiety at all, this may be an unrealistic goal. As the following illustrations show, however, it is very possible to reduce fear and anxiety to a manageable level.

> Kate had become a fearful flyer as an adult and eventually enrolled on a fear of flying course. She now flies when necessary, and appreciates the fact that she no longer spends the days before a holiday dreading the flight and can enjoy being away without worrying about flying home. She still gets slightly anxious at the airport and during take-off, but reminds herself that she enjoys holidays once she arrives and uses the relaxation techniques she was taught on the course.

Most people find that they have to keep using the techniques which have worked to reduce their fear, although often these become so 'automatic' that they don't require much effort.

> Paul started to avoid flying after being very frightened when his flight home from Florida encountered turbulence. He consulted a psychologist who taught him some techniques for controlling his anxious thoughts, similar to those contained in Chapter 7 of this book. Several years later, Paul was woken up when his overnight flight encountered turbulence. It wasn't until he was calmly eating breakfast that he realized he'd been almost unconsciously using the techniques he'd been taught.

It is possible to reduce your fear and anxiety when flying and the information and techniques in this book are a good start. Flying may never be your favourite way to travel, but there are many ways to make it bearable enough that you can fly when you need to. This is the aim of the rest of this book.

## How do psychological techniques overcome fear of flying?

Through our extensive experience, we have learnt that most people who are motivated to overcome their fear of flying are held back by their thoughts and reactions to and about flying, and not just by their knowledge about flight safety. We know that a sizeable proportion of fearful flyers have almost encyclopaedic knowledge about flight safety. However, they find that this insight and knowledge does little to help quell their catastrophizing thoughts and unpleasant, seemingly uncontrollable, physical reactions.

Giving reassuring statistics to those who come for treatment with fears and phobias may therefore not help them to overcome their fear. Many people who seek help already know these facts. Instead, psychologists who work with fearful flyers have recently turned their attention to looking at how to cope with the irrational aspect of people's fears and to devising ways in which such people can manage those feared situations more positively. There are several ways in which targeted psychological therapy (such as cognitive behavioural therapy) can help you to overcome this specific fear, and this is the model adopted in this book:

- **Education.** Factual information about anxiety, fears and phobias will help you to overcome the problem. Such information is included in this book, together with advice on how to decide if it's appropriate for you and how to use it. We also include a section on flight, flight safety and turbulence, as questions about some of these are commonly asked by people we treat.
- **Verbal discussion.** Psychological therapy is designed to help you to overcome specific personal problems. First, though, the therapist must listen carefully to what is bothering you the most. This is achieved by engaging in a sympathetic manner with you and asking you many questions to help to understand and clarify your specific problem. If you have a fear of flying, this enquiry should centre on your fear. If you are asked umpteen questions about your early childhood and upbringing and very few about your fear of flying, you might be with the wrong person or in the wrong place! Psychologists have found that insight on its own may not produce changes in your behaviour, and this limitation has been demonstrated in treating a fear of flying. But by the end of the first session, you should feel that you have been listened to and understood. This is the basis for designing a programme to help you to overcome this

very treatable fear. Obviously, this book will not take part in a verbal discussion with you. It does, however, provide you with the tools to begin to understand your own fear and to select the psychological methods most likely to help you. The contents of this book reflect what we have 'listened to' with hundreds of other fearful flyers and we hope that much of the content is relevant to your specific fear.

- **Challenging ideas and beliefs**. It is important that you learn to see your problem differently. To help to achieve this, we will explain how anxiety affects you and what you can do to overcome the symptoms. Psychologists typically work with you to plan mini experiments which are designed to challenge your beliefs and experience of the problem. This book will point you in the right direction to start doing this for yourself.

- **Addressing your worst fears about having this problem**. We will try to make it feel safe to explore some of your fears, whether about the effects of turbulence or a fear of dying. We will encourage and support you in thinking about these and also gradually expose you to some aspects of your fear in order to improve your confidence and coping skills. Working through this book will help you identify the worst aspects of your fear and teach you some helpful techniques to improve your coping skills.

- **Challenging your safety behaviours**. These are rituals, habits or other ways of behaving that make you feel safer, for example, avoiding flying completely. They may, however, be preventing you from making good progress even though they are protecting you from the situations that expose you to what you fear. This book will help you recognize your own safety behaviours and start to change them.

- **Homework tasks**. A lot of change happens because of things you can do on your own. The 'Stop and Think' exercises in this book are designed to act in a similar way to homework tasks.

In modern psychology, cognitive behavioural therapy is often used to help understand and to teach skills and ideas for overcoming certain problems. Cognitive behavioural therapy has been developed through extensive research and is often used by psychologists to treat fears and anxieties. It is also endorsed by doctors as being safe and effective. It is particularly useful for overcoming a fear of flying because it links how you think about the problem to the way in which you react to it. This is often what drives anxious thoughts and feelings and unhelpful behaviour.

A small word of caution: you may need to be patient with this process and with your rate of progress, because experience shows that lasting change is gradual and incremental. It is almost unheard of for someone who has struggled with a fear of flying and who receives treatment to suddenly stand up and say, 'I have been so silly about having this problem. Of course I was making a big fuss all along. Now where's the boarding gate!?' It is much more likely that you will gain confidence and improve your skills over a period of time. Our job is to help make that happen as quickly as possible. But it is also to help you to do so in a way that is based on tried and tested psychological techniques.

## A case study of one fearful flyer

Now that we have introduced the techniques employed in this book, we'll look at a more detailed case study than those in Chapter 2. As before, we have changed any personal details, but Judith's story is a very good illustration of one person's experience of being afraid to fly and the way in which the techniques in this book helped her overcome her fear. When you read it, you will see how the techniques which were effective for Judith were those which, together with a psychologist, she identified as most useful to overcoming her own unique fear. Judith's experience will not be an exact match to your own but it is a valuable illustration of how to apply the skills and techniques included in this book:

Judith had always been anxious about flying and would only travel with her partner. Judith was convinced that if she travelled on her own she would become so fearful that she would be unable to cope. She described the thought of becoming anxious while travelling alone as 'unbearable', as fear would make her feel physically ill. Judith's partner was occasionally able to persuade her to fly and would spend the flight offering constant reassurance. This limited the number of holidays they could share and where they could travel to and also put their relationship under strain when any conversation about flying came up. When she was promoted to a senior marketing role in her company which would mean travelling around Europe to give presentations, Judith decided to 'sort herself out' and enrolled on a one-day fear of flying course.

The course went well and Judith found that she was even able to relax and walk around a little in the group flight which took place in the second half of the day. She recalls feeling that the flight was a team effort as 'everyone was in it together'. The next week, Judith flew to Edinburgh to give an important presentation. She used some of the techniques taught on the course and spent both flights reading a book she had been looking forward to. As she settled into her new professional role, Judith became more confident about flying and even surprised her partner by booking a weekend in Europe.

Three years later, Judith's mother, who lived in Scotland, became ill and Judith became part of the family 'care team', flying to Scotland every third weekend. Although her partner was very supportive, Judith started to dread the Fridays when she would go straight to the airport after work, flying home late on Sunday after a stressful and strenuous weekend. Fortunately, after nine very unpleasant months, Judith's mother recovered and her partner proposed a relaxing holiday in the Caribbean.

Driving to the airport for their holiday, Judith began to feel very anxious about the flight and was convinced that she would panic in the aircraft. By the time they reached the departure gate she was in tears and it took all the reassurance her partner could offer to persuade her to get on the flight. Although she tried all the techniques from the course which she could remember, Judith did panic when the flight encountered turbulence and her partner had to ask some of the cabin crew for help to stop her hyperventilating. When they landed, Judith vowed to organize a sea journey to return home. As this was not possible, she spent the holiday worrying about the return flight and eventually persuaded a local doctor to prescribe medication for use on the flight. She slept for most of the flight home and resolved to avoid flying whenever possible.

When she returned to work, Judith found that a major presentation had been scheduled in Amsterdam in three months' time and that flights had been booked in her absence. Both she and her partner were distressed at the return of Judith's fear but saw this as an opportunity to seek more specialist help for her fear of flying. Judith consulted her GP, who in turn referred her to a psychologist.

Judith wanted to be able to travel for leisure and professional reasons whenever she needed to. She wanted to be free of the anxiety she experienced whenever she thought about or discussed flying. She also wanted to be able to travel without having to rely on her partner but felt too afraid to even contemplate this possibility. Judith didn't think that flying would ever be an experience to enjoy, but she wanted to be confident enough to fly to long-haul destinations on holiday and travel as was required for her work.

The psychologist first explained to her how therapy could help her. He told her that it was important to understand more about her specific thoughts about her fear as well as how it affected her feelings and behaviours, as people could be affected in different ways. This was an eye-opener for her; she had previously assumed that everyone who had a fear of flying had the same fear and needed identical help in order to overcome their fear. In her therapy, she and her psychologist looked back at the one-day fear of flying course she had done previously to see which aspects of the course had been helpful and which hadn't. Working with the psychologist, Judith realized that she probably did have a phobia of flying and that the main focus of her anxiety was 'fear of fear'. In other words, she was most fearful of the physical symptoms of her fear, which she found very distressing. Information on what causes the physical sensations of anxiety (you can find similar information in Chapter 5 of this book) helped Judith begin to understand more about the way in which her anxiety relating to flying specifically affected her.

As she and the psychologist explored her fear of flying, Judith began to identify some of the factors which may have contributed to her fear. In particular, she understood that the stress of caring for and worrying about her mother may have helped her previous anxieties to re-emerge, and may even have reinforced them. The experience of panicking during her holiday flight also contributed to a fear of being fearful or panicking. A vicious cycle had been created.

Working with the psychologist, Judith also began to explore why taking a fear of flying course had not permanently removed her fear. She was able to recognize that taking a flight specially designed as part of a course, with a group who all felt anxious and with staff who were there to help, can be very different from travelling alone. During the course, so much information was offered that she couldn't focus too much on worrying about becoming afraid. The flight was over so quickly and was so busy that she didn't pay attention to how she felt. The group session had not helped her to realize how anxious she would become about 'being afraid'.

Judith began to realize that feeling anxious or afraid is uncomfortable and unpleasant but not dangerous. The psychologist helped her realize this by talking about fear and anxiety (similar information can be found in Chapter 4 of this book). He also worked with Judith to establish that none of her previous experiences of anxiety had actually caused her any harm, although they had been very unpleasant. Judith also learnt and practised relaxation techniques to help reduce some of the physical symptoms of anxiety (such techniques can be found in Chapter 8). The psychologist accompanied her on a short return 'practice' flight and Judith's presentation in Amsterdam won a major sales contract.

The rest of this book contains information which will enable you to better understand your fear of flying and to change your thoughts and behaviours. Some of this can be used to educate yourself about fear and anxiety or about the technical and safety aspects of flying, if that is an appropriate approach for you. The next two chapters start this process by helping you to understand what causes and maintains a fear of flying.

# 4

# Understanding your fear of flying

Fear of flying is similar to other types of anxiety and needs to be treated accordingly. No matter how many times your friends or colleagues tell you that 'flying is much safer than driving a car', you may still not feel convinced. If anything, such comments may lead you to feel even more distressed and self-conscious about your fear. Although the statistics show that flying is many times safer than any other mode of transport, this knowledge alone is unlikely to help you overcome your fear. Instead, it is an enhanced understanding of your anxiety and advice on how to deal with your flying anxiety, combined with a technical and statistical knowledge of flying, that can help you conquer your fears.

Technically, a fear of flying is a specific type of anxiety disorder. Anxiety affects your body, your thoughts and your actions. It is usually accompanied by a sense that something awful is about to happen. You may think that travelling on a plane will lead to something awful happening to you, that you could lose control or make a complete fool of yourself in front of strangers.

### Maria, aged 40

I was fine until the turbulence started. They switched the seat-belt sign on and I felt a jolt in my stomach. Here we go ... shaking from side to side and up and down. The captain made an announcement asking the cabin crew to sit down. At that point I began shaking like a leaf. Surely it must be serious if the crew are having to sit down? I scrutinize the lovely girl who served me my apple juice earlier. Is there any sign of fear on her face? Does she know something that I don't? I don't feel safe; what if the pilots lose control of the aircraft? Will I be able to get out? I try to talk to the person next to me but he is fully occupied by the in-flight movie. I am so hot that I think my skin will start burning soon. I use the airline magazine to fan myself. Another shake of the aircraft – this time I scream. People are turning around, looking at me. Oh no – I'm so embarrassed. Then, to my utter disbelief, the shaking stops and the cabin crew resume their duties. Phew ... I completed yet another journey on the plane. I am better than I used to be.

Maria's story illustrates common worries that are likely to enter the mind of a fearful flyer: fear of losing control, making a fool of oneself or being trapped in between other passengers. It is Maria's worry that leads her to act in a certain way during turbulence – scanning the faces of the cabin crew for signs of fear, fanning herself down with the aircraft magazine and gasping while trying to suppress her screams. Despite feeling uncomfortable before and during the flight, Maria is able to complete her journey. This brings her a step closer to beating her fear. When Maria first sought help from a psychologist, she had avoided air travel for the past six years after having experienced turbulence on a flight to Japan. Since then she has managed to confront her fear and has completed two short-haul journeys within Europe. Maria's next challenge is a long-haul trip to the United States with her family.

Fear is the normal response to perceived danger or stress, though like many phobias, a fear of flying is not regarded as a rational one, as we will explain. It becomes a psychological problem when it is out of proportion, prevents us from doing things which we can achieve or goes on for too long. For a few, it may be linked to a traumatic flying experience, while for others it can develop 'out of the blue'. Once people develop a fear of flying they may be exposed to a number of unpleasant effects. These include bodily or physical symptoms as well as changes in the way they think, feel and behave. Unless these changes are managed, he or she may 'spin out of control', causing increased fear, discomfort and anxiety. The person may then worry about flying and become anxious about experiencing the unpleasant effects and symptoms of fear. These unfortunately mutually reinforce one another. This can then lead to a panic attack. When this occurs, there is often a sense of hopelessness, which gives rise to the question: 'Will I ever overcome my fear of flying?' But despite the doubt, the majority of people who seek treatment have successfully managed to beat their fear.

## Physical or bodily signs of anxiety

Most people who have a fear of flying recognize the unpleasant physical signs of 'stress', 'worry', 'anxiety' or 'nerves'. Just experiencing them can also make you feel upset, frightened or even desperate. Some of the physical signs of anxiety can mimic physical or mental illness, which can be all the more frightening and makes things feel even worse. Psychologists who help to treat people suffering from fears and anxiety recognize that the physical symptoms can trigger an increase in fear, which only makes the symptoms worse. This is what happens when people suffer a panic attack. The physical or bodily signs that are associated with fear generally, and with a fear of flying specifically, include the following:

- shortness of breath; rapid breathing and panting
- pounding heart
- dry mouth; difficulty swallowing
- sweating
- feeling dizzy or faint
- nausea; feeling ill; bowel discomfort or an urgent need to visit the toilet
- shakiness and trembling, especially in the hands and legs
- headache, muscle aches and pains
- feeling tired.

If others are travelling with the person they may notice that their anxious companion yawns a lot, has stooped posture, clenches his or her jaw and fists and has become very uncommunicative. At best, the person may become repetitive in his or her speech and say the same thing over and over (e.g. 'I don't want to do this', 'We are all going to die'), reduce conversation to few or single words (e.g. 'No', 'Leave me alone') or may withdraw completely and say nothing at all.

Prolonged anxiety states can also affect a person's physical health. Certain physical health problems may be related to psychological difficulties, and these are termed 'psychosomatic problems'. The most common psychosomatic problems associated with general anxiety are breathing difficulties and asthma, skin conditions such as eczema and psoriasis, and high blood pressure due to stress. These conditions can be managed by treating the symptoms as well as the underlying anxiety.

Some passengers who feel anxious may act aggressively towards those around them, including travelling companions as well as strangers. Fearful flyers need to take care that they do not leave their fears unchecked by avoiding seeking professional help if they have difficulty managing their anxiety; a few have inadvertently become aggressive on board aircraft and have been charged with air rage offences. The use of alcohol or certain illicit drugs taken to quell 'nerves' can increase aggression.

## What makes fears and phobias unique?

In terms of psychological difficulties, fears and phobias are both similar to and in some ways different from other problems such as low mood (depression), stress or eating problems. Here are some ways in which the experience of anxiety and phobias is unique:

- The effects are often immediate; the signs and symptoms can creep up unnoticed and become overwhelming in a very short space of time.
- The intensity of these immediate symptoms can often present as a medical emergency, requiring psychological and medical intervention to cope with them.
- Both the mind and body are often affected and this too can make us feel overwhelmed, in turn increasing our anxiety – this effect can produce a panic attack.
- They are among the most treatable psychological problems and so relief from their effects should not be far away if we seek appropriate help.

Phobias are intense fears which arise in certain situations only, but may not be present in others. For example, a person may be able to cope with short-haul flights, but long-haul flights that involve crossing continents may be too difficult for him or her to bear. Phobias typically lead to avoidance of the situations that we fear because we know that our anxiety will increase if we have to deal with these situations. Avoidance only makes the phobia worse, because we quickly build up a defensive story about why we can't do whatever it is we fear. Life then becomes a series of rituals designed to make us feel safer (these are termed 'safety behaviours') and it may be dominated by attempts to avoid the situation we fear.

Below is a list of many of the fears that people talk about when they seek professional help to overcome their fear of flying:

- heights;
- enclosed spaces;
- feeling out of control of how they and others may react;
- the physical sensations of being on a plane (e.g. turbulence, turning, engine sounds);
- lack of familiarity with how planes actually fly (and the risk that they may crash);
- disaster scenarios and death;
- air sickness and feeling physically unwell;
- being separated from loved ones (and one's luggage);

- fear of the symptoms of fear (increased heart rate, rapid breathing, feeling that a panic attack is imminent);
- worry that bad feelings experienced on a previous flight will recur;
- not knowing the answer to pressing 'what if …?' questions. Also being afraid to ask them for fear of ridicule;
- emotions and feelings becoming unsettled as a result of taking a flight, making the person more vulnerable to anxiety and depression;
- fear of being in unfamiliar and foreign places;
- fear of leaving home;
- fear of being in very close proximity to strangers.

In order to understand more about how fear of flying might affect you, we first need to look at how people are affected generally by anxiety, fears and phobias. Since fear of flying is a form of anxiety, this understanding will help us to gain insight into what we may feel when we start to think negatively about flying.

## Anxiety, fears and phobias

Everyone experiences fear and anxiety at some time; these are normal reactions to certain situations, although people may experience them differently. In fact, anxiety is useful and at times potentially life preserving, so it might be dangerous if we did not experience some anxiety in certain situations. Anxiety helps send messages to the brain that rapidly prompt us to escape from threatening situations, such as an encounter with a dangerous animal or threatening person. Almost everyone experiences some anxiety before doing something for the first time or in situations in which we fear we could possibly let ourselves down, such as going on a first date, having to give a speech at work or at a wedding, sitting down to an exam or attending a job interview. Some anxiety, psychologists have argued, helps us to perform better than if we had no anxiety at all.

Too much anxiety or anxiety that carries on for a long time, however, may become overwhelming and can interfere with our ability to cope or to perform. This is true of air travel; as we saw in Chapter 3, some anxiety about flying is normal and in fact very common. But too much worry, either before you fly or while flying, may affect your enjoyment and comfort, as well as your ability to cope with the flying experience. As we have also seen, some people feel so overwhelmed by their anxiety that they choose to avoid situations where they may encounter its unpleasant effects. That is why so many people who fear flying avoid having to travel by plane wherever they possibly can.

## Unhealthy and healthy forms of anxiety

Let us consider the distinction between fear and anxiety. Imagine that you are crossing the road when all of a sudden a car hits the kerb when turning the corner, causing the driver to lose control. There is a good reason to be afraid. This is fear, because there is an actual threat of injury or serious damage to one's life. Once fear is generated, the brain automatically signals for adrenaline to be released into the body, which activates our general arousal system. This biological process ensures physical arousal, helping the body to prepare for dealing with threatening situations. The main effect is to increase our heart rate so that blood can be rapidly pumped to the main muscles that help us to escape, mainly to our legs and arms.

When the fear is intense enough our animal-like instincts take over. This will often cause a person to respond to a critical event in one of three ways – known as the fight-flight-freeze responses – or in a combination of these. It is easy to see how the flight response may be crucial for escaping from the threat of being hit by a speeding car. Equally plausible is the idea that the driver may avoid hitting the pedestrian by actively fighting to regain control of the car. What may be less obvious is the way in which the freeze response is just as basic. The sound of the car hitting the kerb may cause you to become temporarily immobilized. Your legs may feel as if they are glued to the pavement and you are unable to move in either direction. This may alert the driver to your exact presence, thereby making it easier for him or her to manoeuvre the car away from you. Fear is a healthy response to danger that can be crucial for human (and animal) survival.

However, if you are worried about being hit by a car every time you cross the road, whether or not cars are in sight, anxiety has become an irrational fear. Anxiety is often not helpful because the threat is imaginary. It is therefore likely that you are wasting a lot of energy and time on worrying about what might – but not necessarily will – happen. This is not to say that there are no risks involved in crossing the road. In fact, there is some risk involved in everything that we do, whether it is gardening or travelling on the bus to work. A problem can arise when the probability of danger attached to any given situation is unnecessarily overestimated. This can cause us to become increasingly fearful, to the extent that we start to avoid doing the things we wish to do. This happened to Sarah, who decided to resign from work because of her fear.

Sarah worked as a bank manager in the City and had been using public transport for the past ten years. Over the past six months, Sarah had become increasingly anxious during her travels to and from work. Symptoms included dizziness, nausea, tension and sleep difficulties. She began to call in sick at work, thinking that she just needed some time away from the pressure of working in the banking industry. This made her worries even worse, as she would spend a great deal of time contemplating the various dangers that might occur once she began travelling to work again. Sarah loved her job but felt that the strains of the commute were too difficult to bear. She eventually resigned from her job in the City and began working for a charity in her local area.

## Understanding your own fear of flying

One way to better understand your own fear of flying is to ask yourself whether you tend to be anxious in other situations that do not necessarily involve flying. Sometimes anxiety seems to go on and on and can become a lifelong problem. There can be a number of reasons for this. Some people may have an anxious personality or have 'learnt' to worry. Others may have a series of stressful life events to cope with, for example bereavements, redundancy or divorce. Yet others may be under pressure, at work or at home, because of family problems or financial difficulties.

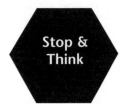

**Stop & Think**

How often do you feel anxious (often, rarely, sometimes, never)? What kinds of situations are most likely to make you feel anxious (meeting new people, stress at work, encounters with certain objects/animals, health problems, finances, etc.)? How long does your anxiety last (weeks, days, hours, minutes)? Is there a pattern to your anxiety (does it occur on a specific day, in a specific context or a particular time of the year/day)? How does anxiety affect you (eating, sleeping, concentration, memory, sex drive, energy, motivation, etc.)?

People who have a fear of flying often say they are convinced something 'bad' will happen if they fly. While it can make you feel uncomfortable, fear is rarely dangerous – even if your mind and body are telling you otherwise. It is important to recognize that each person is unique; what is perceived as 'threatening' for one flyer may not necessarily be the same for another. This can be reassuring in itself; no two fearful flyers are exactly alike. It means that we might be able to ask, 'Why do other people seem to cope with their fear?'

A deeper understanding about the nature of anxiety and fear, as well as phobias, is useful in order to gain insight into how you think and feel about air travel. This paves the way for explaining how to overcome your fear of flying. What causes people to develop a fear of flying in the first place? This fundamental question is addressed in the next chapter.

# 5

# What causes your fear of flying?

As we saw in the previous chapter, people who fear flying do so for a variety of reasons. Some feel claustrophobic on board an aircraft. Others fear heights. Many have an intense dislike of turbulence and express extreme fear that they will become injured, or even worse, as a result of this. Some passengers have difficulty coping with 'disrupted attachments'; they don't like to be separated from loved ones or their baggage. Fear of the unknown and heightened anxiety about not being in control are also often expressed by people who fear flying. People may worry about how they will react and whether they can cope with their own feelings, such as anxiety and panic, if they become emotionally distressed while flying.

A surprisingly large number of people also worry about how others will cope. For example, parents may express concern that their child may become terrified and inconsolable. Others may worry about the possible reactions of a travelling companion or partner. The effects of jet lag, altitude, low humidity in the cabin and stress of air travel can also interact with prescribed medications to make some passengers feel especially vulnerable and out of control, and may trigger feelings of anxiety. Some find being abroad or in close proximity to strangers particularly difficult to contend with. As you can see, there are probably as many different causes of fear of flying as there are people who dislike flying!

## Identifying individual triggers

What triggers flying anxiety in the first place? What sets off the internal alarm, like the siren on an ambulance or a police car? These are questions which often preoccupy fearful flyers. For some, the fear can initially 'come out of the blue'. The first anxiety attack may be completely unexpected and appear not to be triggered by anything. If this was true for you, try to remember the first time you experienced a fear of flying:

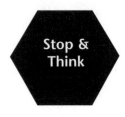

Stop &
Think

Was there anything else happening in your life at the same time you first experienced a fear of flying? Were you feeling stressed because of work or a relationship problem? Did you undergo a major change in your life circumstances at the same time that your fear of flying came about? Look back over the last few months to see if anything unsettled you in a significant way.

It is important to recognize that what triggered an anxiety attack in the first place may not be completely obvious. But most often, careful analysis of what went on in your life often reveals that there was in fact a trigger, even if it was not the one that you immediately thought about. These are some of the factors which may be responsible for triggering flying-related anxiety:

• feeling tense before or during a flight, for whatever reason;
• other emotional states, such as worry, anger, grief, or a sense of sadness, which may cause bodily reactions before and/or during the flight;
• other changes in your physical state caused, for example, by illness or excessive tiredness;
• the effects of certain drugs and/or alcohol, or other more immediate triggers, such as low blood sugar, jet lag or being stuck in a traffic jam in a car on your way to the airport.

Some people can identify particular situations which appear to have caused the fear of flying in the first place. These triggers tend to vary from one fearful flyer to another, but it is possible to distinguish between two common types of causes. The first type is a direct experience of an uncomfortable or frightening situation. This includes being stuck on board a plane during a delay due to bad weather or an air traffic hold-up, resulting in feeling trapped, which is termed 'claustrophobia'. Other triggers include encountering turbulence or bad weather while in flight; a flashback to a memory of an incident where you fainted or maybe even vomited in front of other passengers; a minor technical fault on the aircraft; and unpleasant experiences with airline staff during check-in and security procedures prior to flying. The second type is indirect exposure, for example through seeing media reports of an air crash or documentaries about aircraft accidents or crashes, watching movies that involve injury or death in an air crash or listening to the stories of someone who has had a bad flying experience. Being around others who are afraid of flying can also trigger flying anxiety. This may occur when a child acquires the anxiety from a parent.

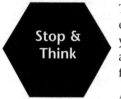

Try to think about the first time you experienced fear of flying. What happened before you arrived at the airport? Can you think of any event that may have contributed to your fear of flying?

Although it can be helpful to try and find out what it was that initially triggered your fear of flying, don't get too preoccupied with it and don't worry if you cannot find a clear explanation for your fear. It may be more helpful to focus your efforts on learning how to cope with your anxiety, even if you do not know what triggered it in the first place.

## The effects of flying on your body

It may be helpful to know that the experience of flying can increase fear in susceptible people because of the effects flying has on the body. Flying involves challenge within our bodies, because of the way in which the environment in an aircraft cabin differs from the normal experience of being on the ground. The human body was clearly not designed for being an airline passenger and we sometimes react to the cabin environment in ways that increase fear and anxiety. The three main physical and mental effects are motion sickness, disorientation and mild lack of oxygen. There are effective techniques you can use to help with each of these, and we will describe them in Chapter 7. This section describes each of these effects, in order to help build your understanding of what might be causing your own fear of flying.

### Motion sickness and disorientation

Research shows that people who are anxious about flying tend to suffer from motion sickness more frequently than those who are not anxious. Motion sickness and disorientation both happen to a proportion of people when flying because of the way in which our sight, sense of balance and sensations of movement interact. They also occur because fear can result in an increase of adrenaline flowing around the body; the prolonged effects can upset the stomach, making us feel nauseated and/or giving rise to an urgent need to visit the toilet. Because aircraft move in three dimensions we often receive conflicting signals which our brains find disorientating. This is what leads to disorientation or sickness. Disorientation and motion sickness are unpleasant and on their own will often increase the anxiety associated with flying. They also reduce your ability to think clearly, making it harder to manage your anxiety. (This is one reason why we suggest that you don't plan to do any demanding or important work even on long flights – it may not be a realistic aim.)

If you associate flying with feeling unwell, you are, quite reasonably, likely to become anxious when thinking about taking a flight. You don't have to feel unwell or actually vomit to start to associate flying with motion sickness. Very low levels of motion sickness are possibly enough to stimulate anxiety about air travel. If this might be you, take the time to talk to your doctor or pharmacist about the effective remedies available and make sure you use them whenever you fly.

The important thing to understand is that the three-dimensional movement of aircraft can contribute to motion sickness and disorientation, which can increase anxiety and reduce your ability to think clearly. If you'd like to know more about how this happens, here's a further explanation.

You have a very sophisticated system built into each ear which detects whether you are upright and which way your head is moving (for those of you who have done or use some biology, this is the vestibular system). When you are sitting in an aircraft which rolls to the right to start a turn, your balance system will detect this and your eyes and balance system will both tell you that the aircraft is turning right. If the aircraft stays in the turn for more than a few seconds and then rolls to the left to fly straight again, your balance system may not detect that the aircraft is flying straight. Instead, it may signal to your brain that you are turning left. Now your eyes tell you that you are flying straight and your ears signal that you are turning left. This leads to disorientation and can feel very unpleasant.

As a rule of thumb, if you think that you are becoming disorientated, try and concentrate on what your sight tells you is happening. Keep looking ahead, not down at your feet! This is how pilots are trained to deal with situations like this. Your body will quite quickly make sense of the conflicting signals and you will not feel disorientated for very long. Combined with relaxing breathing (as explained in Chapter 8), this is a very effective way of dealing with motion sickness and disorientation.

### The cabin environment

The environment in an aircraft cabin is similar to that you would find at approximately 8,000 feet above sea level if you climbed a mountain.

Because of this, the pressure of oxygen available is slightly lower than most people are used to. This is not dangerous to healthy people but it is one of the reasons why doctors occasionally suggest that people with certain medical conditions breathe additional oxygen when they fly. The very slight decrease in the level of oxygen in your blood may cause your body to react in ways that are very similar to the bodily sensations of anxiety we described in the previous chapter: you may have an increased heart rate or tend to breathe more rapidly. Because this is very similar to the physical sensations of anxiety, it may be interpreted as fear rather than the body responding to the cabin environment. If this happens, we are often pre-programmed to think 'if I am feeling anxious, this must be dangerous', and anxiety and fear can begin to increase rapidly. If you think this might be happening to you, there are some techniques in Chapter 7 which can help.

## Lack of control

Fear of flying isn't really about the risks inherent in aviation. Instead it is based on the uncomfortable awareness that life is fragile and vulnerable and that none of us – despite our best efforts – has complete control of it. This applies to most of us, whether in the air or on the ground. John, for example, felt very vulnerable on board the aircraft because he was not 'in control' of the plane.

### John, aged 30
I do not have wings and I was not designed to fly like a bird. Then why am I stepping on board this plane? I obviously need to because I can't give in to the fear. I need to be strong and do my best to keep it under control. Of course I want to visit my family abroad – why else would I be trying so hard? I did it last year too, so why is it not getting any easier? Never mind the fact that I squeezed the arm rest so hard that I thought my knuckles would fall off. I bet the old lady next to me thought I was vandalizing airline property. Mind you, the cabin interior is simply not designed for people like me. I am stuck between two gigantic men snoring through the night. What if they don't wake up and I become trapped here for ever? I could never fall asleep – I need to stay alert. For what, though? It's not so much that flying is unnatural ... but when I find myself up in the sky, sealed in the cabin, I feel more vulnerable than anywhere else. I am not flying the plane, I am not in control. Instead my safety and wellbeing has been put in the hands of someone else – the

pilots and the crew. It is a scary prospect but maybe I should learn to trust other people more. Yuck – the thought makes me feel sick!

Many passengers seated in an aircraft worry excessively about the dangers of flight. Despite the safety statistics, they become fixated and disabled by fear and may spend a majority of the flight praying for a safe landing. Their minds may be plagued by the terror of a dozen catastrophic scenarios. These tend to have one thing in common: worrying thoughts that are concerned with what might happen as opposed to what is actually happening. What if the aircraft falls from the sky? What if I end up being sick on other passengers during turbulence? What if I am not able to cope during the flight? What if the equipment on board the aircraft is not working? Why is there condensation coming from the air conditioning system? What is that smell? What will these terrifying minutes feel like as the plane plunges to earth before crashing? These are just a few of the many thoughts possibly circulating around the mind of a fearful flyer. Even though none of us is ever in total control of all of these issues, we can all learn to be in command of our thoughts and feelings.

## Worrying thoughts

When we fear something, such as flying, we may have exaggerated, distorted or unpleasant thoughts and feelings about things or situations. These tend to be negative and reflect also our fears about how and why we might not cope. They range from mild apprehension, such as 'I'm not sure that I will cope very well with the flight', to extreme fears, such as 'I will die if I have to go on that thing'. These feelings may dent our confidence, lower our mood and make us feel negative, vulnerable, depressed and even out of control. Psychologists[1] have identified a number of common thought patterns, or 'thinking errors', that reflect and maintain negative emotions. The ten most common ones are:

1  **All-or-nothing thinking**: a tendency to think in absolute or extreme terms about a situation, mostly in a negative way. For example: 'Flying is always very risky' or 'I could never enjoy flying'.
2  **Over-generalization**: the use of individual cases to build up a picture that generates a (usually false) rule. For example: 'The fact that the plane crash-landed at Heathrow means that you can never feel completely safe flying.' This discounts other relevant information, such as the fact that everyone on board the aircraft survived

---

[1]   Burns, D. (2000). *The Feeling Good Handbook*, 2nd edition. USA: Plume.

and only a handful of people had any injuries. Another might be: 'The flight attendant looks really serious; something bad must be happening.'

3  **Mental filter**: focusing on negative or upsetting experiences or thoughts while ignoring other aspects that paint a different picture of the situation. For example: 'Turbulence is dangerous and the plane is going to crash.' The facts are that a large number of flights encounter some air turbulence and aircraft are built to withstand it, but this important information is ignored or discounted.

4  **Disqualifying the positive**: discounting positive experiences because you do not seem to want them, or to be able to replace your strongly held pessimistic views or memory of experiences. For example: 'Even though we arrived at our holiday destination safely, there is always the dreaded return journey.'

5  **Jumping to conclusions or mind reading**: a tendency to assume that the worst will happen in spite of a lack of evidence to support it. For example: 'I could have a panic attack and possibly die', in spite of the fact that the two events are hardly linked and that you have not previously suffered a panic attack.

6  **Catastrophizing**: exaggerating the negative characteristics of a situation, however unlikely they are. For example: 'The delay means that there is something wrong with the plane, which they are not telling us about. There is something seriously wrong and we are going to be involved in an accident.'

7  **Emotional reasoning**: making decisions based on how you feel rather than on the facts that explain a situation. For example: 'I feel very anxious. My heart is pounding and I feel faint. Something bad is going to happen on this trip; I just know it.'

8  **Should, must and have-to**: a tendency to distort your thoughts, 'fixing' yourself rigidly in a situation and making yourself seem to be governed by quite extreme or inflexible rules. For example: 'I should be able to cope with this. I shouldn't have any unpleasant feelings. It must be because the pills aren't working. I have to give up my job.' (You may be amused by the slight irreverence of a famous therapist called Albert Ellis, who termed this tendency 'musterbation'.)

9  **Labelling**: this is similar to over-generalization and reflects a tendency to explain events through categorizing, labelling or naming them in fixed terms, rather than by describing them behaviourally. For example: 'It was a plane load of frightened passengers', rather than 'some passengers got worried when they were told that

the flight would need to divert to another airport because of bad weather at our destination.'

10 **Personalization or attribution:** exaggerating causation when facts do not necessarily support this. For example: 'I got up from my seat and the plane started tilting; it must have been because I unbalanced it', when in fact the aircraft was entering into a turn in order to change course which had no connection with anyone's movements on board.

**Stop & Think**

Read through the above thinking errors one more time. See if you can recognize any of them among your own thought process. Make a note of your thoughts. Are you able to link your individual thoughts to any or all of the ten common thinking errors?

Worrying may sometimes reach frightening proportions, leaving you feeling vulnerable. This can lead to a panic attack. The experience of a panic attack only reinforces the sense of dread about flying in addition to the unpleasant physical signs, thoughts and feelings associated with anxiety and panic.

As we have stressed, there are many reasons why people develop fear of flying in the first place. These will often vary from one person to another due to individual differences in bodily reactions, feelings of lacking control and thinking styles, to name a few. This is why we do not find it effective to use a 'one-size-fits-all' approach to treat fears. The next chapter describes the way in which fear of flying is maintained. It is hoped that this will encourage you to break free from the cycles that reinforce your fear.

# 6

# Why can't I reduce my fear of flying even though I keep trying?

Some people whom we have helped have asked: 'What drives or maintains my fear of flying?' This is a good question and the answer may be reassuring and helpful. Anxiety problems come from a distorted belief about the level of danger that we associate with certain situations, bodily sensations or mental events. Once we have experienced anxious feelings, several things can reactivate fear and anxiety. These include:

- the same or similar situations;
- the same or similar feelings, sensations and bodily and mental sensations that we have experienced before;
- catastrophizing about the event or situation, where we fear the worst possible outcome, which simply maintains our high levels of anxiety.

This chapter will help you identify the ways in which your current coping strategies may be part of your flying anxiety. Imagine that you parked your car on a double yellow line and received a parking fine. If you then continued to park on a double yellow line every week, it is likely that the problem of receiving financial penalties would persist. An effective solution to the problem might be to park your car elsewhere, as this would stop the parking officer from repeatedly issuing you with costly parking fines.

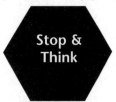

**Stop & Think**

How do you normally cope with fear? Do you escape the situation? Talk yourself out of the fear? Use medication or alcohol? Distract yourself (read, listen to music)? Ask for help (from a friend, talk to your partner/colleague/fellow passenger, etc.)?

We have come across many people who initially thought that they would never be able to fly. We have often found that the behaviours these people used to help themselves cope with fear were the same problematic behaviours that worsened their emotional problems! The experience of many of these people, some of whom have had severe flying anxiety, is both inspirational and encouraging. We are optimistic that almost everyone can learn how to beat their fear in a way similar to Christina.

### Christina, aged 40

I never thought I would be able to overcome my fear. I attended two different courses on fear of flying. I survived the flight simulator but I could not get myself to fly the real thing. I eventually sought help from a psychologist. He was very helpful and taught me how to challenge unhelpful thoughts. I became a master at relaxation skills and I even changed some of my behaviours. I used to think that my 'safety behaviours' were effective ways of keeping me safe. It was a difficult journey but one that changed my life for ever. I think my family and friends were shocked when I completed my first plane trip to Amsterdam. I still get apprehensive about flying but it is nothing like the horrific terror it used to be for me.

## The vicious cycle of flying anxiety

Flying anxiety can affect you in at least four different ways:

- the way you feel;
- the way you think;
- the way you behave;
- the way your body works.

The symptoms you experience may be frightening, particularly if you are not able to identify them merely as signs of anxiety. Table 6.1 lists various symptoms of anxiety. You may wish to highlight those that apply to you.

Anyone who has ever experienced extreme anxiety or a panic attack knows just how unpleasant the experience can be. The experience is stored in the person's memory, leading him or her to avoid any situation that may reawaken these unpleasant feelings. These people come to fear the experience of fear itself. When we develop a fear of fear itself, this is called secondary anxiety. Many people who have a fear of flying also have a fear of the physical and emotional effects of being fearful. This will often cause extreme anxiety, or even panic and an avoidance of flying in the future, because of how unpleasant the thought of flying and anxiety itself are for the person.

For example, someone who has experienced anxiety during a particular flight may start to feel anxious in anticipation of flying and become frightened of the symptoms themselves. This worry can

**Table 6.1 Symptoms of anxiety**

| How you feel | How you think | How you behave | What happens to your body |
|---|---|---|---|
| Anxious, worried, nervous, frightened Tense, stressed, uptight, unsettled Unreal, strange, detached, woozy Panicky | Constant worrying Thoughts racing Imagining the worst and dwelling on it 'I'm losing control' 'The plane will crash' 'I will die' 'I can't cope' 'I can't get out of the plane' 'I'm going to make a fool of myself' 'I am going to faint' | Pace up and down the air terminal Can't sit and relax in the airport lounge Talk quickly or more than usual Be snappy and irritable Drink more Eat more (or less) Avoid airports, flying | Heart pounds, races, skips a beat Stomach churning or butterflies Breathing becomes rapid and shallow Dizzy, light headed Sweating Tense muscles Tingling or numbness in fingers/toes |

actually cause the very symptoms that are feared. The bodily symptoms can, in turn, then reinforce your thoughts, leading you to become even more convinced that something truly awful is going to happen. You may even worry that there is something more seriously wrong with you, especially when other people are seemingly capable of flying without the slightest hint of any worry or concern. This worry can then produce more anxiety symptoms and so a vicious cycle can develop, as illustrated in Figure 6.1.

## Unhelpful coping strategies

How can you break free from the vicious cycle of flying anxiety? When we experience fear, we do not always apply healthy solutions to emotional problems. Therefore, it may feel as if your fear of flying will go on and on despite your best efforts to try to overcome it. You may have already tried some coping techniques, none of which brought you closer to a comfortable flying experience. Certain methods of coping may reflect understandable but unhealthy ways to cope. In particular, they may be used to quell anxiety for a short period of time, but for some people their use simply masks the problem or may even make the effects of anxiety worse.

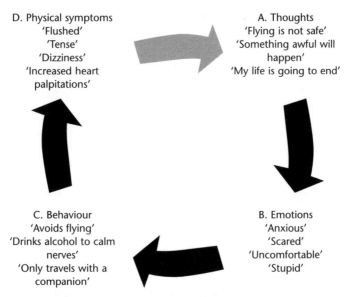

D. Physical symptoms
'Flushed'
'Tense'
'Dizziness'
'Increased heart
palpitations'

A. Thoughts
'Flying is not safe'
'Something awful will
happen'
'My life is going to end'

C. Behaviour
'Avoids flying'
'Drinks alcohol to calm
nerves'
'Only travels with a
companion'

B. Emotions
'Anxious'
'Scared'
'Uncomfortable'
'Stupid'

**Figure 6.1 The vicious cycle of flying anxiety**

Psychologists have recently turned their attention to what maintains our fears as much as what causes them in the first place. There are some common factors that maintain fears and it is important to recognize these and understand how they might affect you if you are to overcome your fear. The following are some examples of unhelpful strategies that you might be using to cope with your flying anxiety.

## Avoidance

Most people seek to escape from stressful situations and do so in a number of different ways. They will avoid situations and feelings that remind them of the unpleasantness that they associate with their fear. It is easy to understand why avoidance is the main coping mechanism used by people who have a fear of flying.

Once a vicious cycle has developed, with anxious thoughts increasing your fear of flying, avoidance is often used as a way of coping with the fear. It is perfectly normal to try to avoid something that is dangerous, but as flying is not a real danger it is more the fear of the symptoms of anxiety that prevents people from flying. Avoidance of flying can result in a great loss of confidence, which can affect how you feel about yourself. What happens is that we come to avoid the unpleasant thoughts and feelings about flying as much as the actual flight.

Those who are either motivated to overcome their fear, or who come under pressure from their family, friends or work colleagues to fly, will find that making excuses and avoidance are not always appropriate options. (It may also be the realization that there are some destinations where taking a train or boat makes no practical sense.)

## Filtering effects

We may use mental filters when thinking about or in response to situations we fear. These make us 'notice' the bad or unpleasant aspects of a situation more than those that signal success and indicate that we are coping with our fear. For example, we listen eagerly to friends and relatives who return from a trip and tell us how bad or unpleasant it was, perhaps referring to flight delays or bad service on board (forgetting that they arrived home safely), which reinforces our fear that flying is a frightening experience that is best avoided.

### Selective memory

A further point to notice is that our memory is selective and may confirm our worst nightmare scenario, even if this is only a small possibility within a larger story. We then fixate on the negative aspect of the experience. For example, someone might have felt overwhelmed by his anxiety and suffered a panic attack. However unpleasant this might have been, it is likely that he recovered from this and eventually coped. Unfortunately, he has continued to worry about both his fear of flying and his extreme reaction to it. These memories are carefully stored and highlight the negative aspects of flying and how the person was affected.

## Excessive checking

Someone who has experienced a panic attack in the past may 'scan' his or her body several times for signs of another pending panic attack. This is to be vigilant to the possibility that he or she may feel ill, have a panic attack or lose bodily control (fainting, vomiting, inability to breathe properly, etc.). Another fearful flyer may frequently look out of the window to ensure that the engines are working, that the weather looks OK or that the aircraft wings are still attached. The problem is that the more a person checks, the more uncertain he or she will feel. Excessive checking is also time consuming and tiring, and can prevent a person from absorbing the positive aspects of a flight.

## *Negative interpretation of symptoms*

Initial signs or symptoms of anxiety (such as increased heart rate and tightness in the chest) can come to maintain the fear. This is in spite of the fact that many people experience minor changes in their heart rate when they are faced with a relatively unfamiliar situation such as flying (since they are unlikely to do this every day). The body recognizes the newness or unfamiliarity of the situation and prepares us to react in order to cope. These normal bodily signs or reactions can lead such people to mistakenly believe that there is something mentally or physically wrong with them. This may cause them to worry and avoid situations which make them feel uneasy in themselves.

## Seeking reassurance

People with a fear of flying may be constantly asking friends and family questions such as 'Is it safe to fly?', 'Do you think the aircraft could fall from the sky during turbulence?', 'Do you think I will make it to Rome?', 'Are you sure it is a good idea for me to fly?' During the flight they may scrutinize other people's behaviours, facial expressions and body language to ensure that there is no sign of anxiety or discomfort from those around them. Unfortunately, excessively seeking reassurance can lower people's confidence in trusting their own judgement. They may also discount the reassurance they are given, triggering more anxious questions.

## Excessive worry

We may think that by worrying about unpleasant events during a flight, we will be able to prevent those events from happening. For example, we may imagine a number of catastrophic events prior to a flight and make a mental note on how to deal with each of them. Often, these anticipated disasters may be products of our imagined worries rather than probable events. If you find that you are spending too much time concentrating on your worry, you are probably becoming fixated on it. The danger is that you may be reinforcing your anxiety and reducing your capacity to do anything constructive to manage it.

## Excessive use of alcohol

Some people may use alcohol to help them quell their nerves during the flight. However, anxiety often re-emerges as soon as the effect of alcohol wears off. You may end up with the added problem of dehydration and a hangover. In addition, there is the potential to develop a new problem – over-reliance on alcohol every time you fly. This can lead you to attribute your ability to fly to the use of alcohol rather than other skills and techniques. Very occasionally, even certain prescribed medications can have the same unwanted effect, and so it is always advisable to check with your doctor whether certain medications can increase stress and anxiety. Alcohol may seem to be a useful and easily available remedy to anxiety, but it does not help you to solve or overcome the problem. It is worth noting that some passengers have a tendency to become aggressive (rather than relaxed) if they consume too much alcohol on board the aircraft. This can adversely affect their behaviour and lead to the unwanted attention of the crew, or worse.

## Specific behaviours or rituals

Most people have rituals in their lives that help them to cope with stressful situations, whether these include wearing a specific item of clothing, saying certain things to themselves in their mind, prayer or mental images that they conjure up to make them feel safe. This is normal and can help people to cope with and overcome difficult and stressful situations. People with a fear of flying may have many such rituals or act in certain ways in order to try to reduce the extent of their fear. For those who do manage to fly – however uncomfortable it is for them psychologically – some will grip their arm rest and endure a 'white knuckle ride' until they are safely back on the ground. Others adopt and rely on specific behaviours or rituals which they believe will make the flight easier to endure by lowering their levels of anxiety and fear. Examples include having a specific seat preference on board the aircraft; restricting their travels to certain airlines or aircraft types; or bringing along an object or token they feel will protect them or distract them from their fears, such as a lucky charm.

Although such rituals can often be helpful, they may be excessive or unnecessary (such as avoiding taking overnight flights in the belief that there is more turbulence at night) and may lead to avoidance. A visit to a psychologist can help you to discover whether the ritual is helpful or unhelpful.

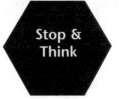

Stop & Think

Note some of the things you have done or would do to make yourself feel safe during a flight. Make a distinction between ordinary safety precautions (e.g. wearing a seat belt for the duration of the flight) and those safety behaviours that prevent you from relaxing (e.g. clutching the arm rest, being overly aware of physical sensations, excessive worry).

Select one safety behaviour that you might like to stop doing. To reduce anxiety you need to reduce these behaviours. This is best done by focusing on each safety behaviour in turn. Ask yourself: is my feared disaster likely to happen if I stop (the specific action you are doing)? Will I feel more relaxed and comfortable if I stop (the specific action you are doing)?

Below is a summary list of behaviours that may help to shine light on why your fear of flying persists or has become worse. It may be a useful exercise to check whether any of these apply to you. A psychologist can also assess whether any of these may be preventing you from overcoming your fear:

- ignoring the problem and not doing anything to confront or overcome it;
- avoidance of flying, not exposing yourself to the situation you fear;
- lack of motivation to overcome the problem;
- over-reliance on safety behaviours and other 'solutions' that may not work;
- getting the wrong sort of help for your problem (e.g. persisting with the idea that the problem comes from something bad that happened to you in your childhood);
- not being helped by what you have tried, but continuing with it anyway;
- applying 'solutions' that are likely to make the problem even worse (e.g. over-reliance on alcohol or certain drugs);
- having other untreated psychological problems that might be 'driving' your fear (e.g. depression, relationship difficulties, alcohol dependency).

Many of the things that we do to cope with our fear can actually maintain the problem. If you recognize any of the behaviours in the list above, it may be worth thinking about other ways to approach your fear of flying. This may require you to challenge anxious thoughts and change unhelpful behaviours. The next chapters provide practical ideas and guidance on how to apply healthy coping strategies that can help you overcome your fear of flying.

# 7

# Practical guidance on managing your fear of flying

The previous chapters introduced the idea of using cognitive behavioural therapy skills to help you to understand the causes and effects of fear of flying. This chapter aims to provide you with much of the information you need in order to start to overcome your fear. As you will have learnt, a fear of flying is not an illness and so can't be cured by a pill. The good news is that modern psychological methods are very effective in helping you overcome this fear. As we described in Chapter 5, a fear of flying affects your body, your mind and your behaviour. As we saw in Chapter 6, when the fear is intense enough, a vicious cycle may occur; our negative thoughts, emotions, behaviours and physical symptoms can start to reinforce one another. This can make the flying anxiety worse. It makes sense to try and deal with these thoughts, emotions, behaviours and symptoms, and to develop targeted skills to overcome the fear.

This chapter describes skills that you can use to make flying less stressful for you. First, we teach you a number of techniques that will allow you to challenge thoughts about imagined and feared catastrophes or disasters. These techniques are particularly appropriate if you notice that your response to the prospect of taking a flight is dominated by anxious or distressing thoughts. Learning how to challenge such thoughts will help you to manage excessive worry, which is often believed to drive anxiety and related safety behaviours. The chapter also provides useful strategies for changing unhelpful behaviours. By avoiding the thing you fear, you may never discover and enjoy the realization that nothing terrible is likely to happen.

You may find some techniques more helpful than others. Don't expect all your fear to disappear straight away: psychologists have found that only by keeping at these skills will you have the best chance of permanently overcoming your fear.

## Learning how to deal with distressing thoughts

We often find that people's expectations can greatly affect their reactions to flying. What people say and do during a flight is largely dependent on how they understand what is happening around them. Some passengers are actually more distressed by their interpretations of flying – the over-focusing on the possible things that could go wrong – than the actual flight itself. You may have experienced light turbulence during a flight and interpreted this as a sign of 'the aircraft being out of control'. It is likely that you felt nervous and you may even have tightened your grip on the arm rest as a natural reaction when in a state of fear, while also hoping that this could somehow ensure a safe flying experience.

The idea that our thinking is linked to our actions and our feelings is the fundamental principle of cognitive behavioural therapy. By understanding your thinking and how it affects your emotions and behaviours, it is possible to develop alternative ways of interpreting your flying experience. The example below illustrates the connection between our thoughts and our reactions.

Lisa was going on holiday to Italy with five of her colleagues from work. She had never been a confident flyer and would always travel with a family member who was familiar with her problem. Lisa met her colleagues at the airport and noticed that she felt anxious and nervous (*emotions*). She silently whispered to herself, 'How will they react when they see that I am anxious? I will make a complete fool of myself' (*thoughts*). No matter how hard she tried to steady her hands, she noticed that they were trembling when passing through security (*physical symptoms*). During take-off Lisa was convinced her colleagues could see that she was shaking (*interpretation*). Once the captain had turned off the seat-belt signs, she quickly got out of her seat and walked down towards the galley area where the crew were preparing the drinks trolley. She did not dare sit next to her colleagues. She explained to the crew that she was a nervous flyer and asked if she was allowed to stand up for the duration of the flight (*behaviour*). Lisa remembered thinking that it was her actions (*avoidance*) that would 'save' her from the expected embarrassment and shame once her colleagues discovered her flaws. She later learnt that her expectations had been unduly pessimistic when her colleagues showed support and empathy during the lead-up to the return flight (*reinterpretation*). Lisa felt an immediate relief and her anxiety level rapidly decreased (*physical and emotional symptoms*).

We now turn to look at your own ideas about flying. Are they unrealistic and unhelpful? Are they likely to help you overcome your fear or are they actually preventing progress? Our thoughts are not always realistic and it is therefore a good idea to look at them. Let's start by identifying your main thoughts about flying. Discovering your key thoughts can be more difficult than you think. They are, more often than not, automatic thoughts that reside in your mind. You may not be conscious of them because you are either so used to them or very good at suppressing them. A good way to identify unhelpful thoughts is to pay attention to emotional changes and use these as a cue for paying attention to your thinking. If you notice any anxiety or tension when you think about flying, for example, stop whatever you are doing (if possible) and ask yourself, 'What am I thinking about right now?'

To start with, identify three or four thoughts that worry you most about flying and make a note of them. The next step is to use the information in this book to check how realistic the thoughts are. Chapter 9 is most likely to help you with this as it provides useful guidance on the technical aspects of flying. If the thoughts that make you anxious are unrealistic, then use the technique that follows to challenge them and replace them with a more helpful way of thinking. The following is a list of examples. You may have other irrational thoughts and it is important that you try and identify each of these. Make a list of your own irrational thoughts, including those below if they apply to you:

*Turbulence is dangerous.*
*Flying is not safe.*
*I won't be able to get out of the plane – I am stuck.*
*Something awful is going to happen to me.*
*I don't feel good – there must be something wrong.*

Everyone with a fear of flying has different ideas about flying, some of which may be similar to your own. If you don't challenge these ideas, you will inevitably be afraid because you assume they are accurate. The rationale for the techniques given here is that selecting and practising an appropriate way of managing or even countering distressing thoughts breaks into the vicious cycle and will therefore help to manage your anxiety and reduce distress.

Suppose you were convinced that turbulence is dangerous. In other words, you believe something bad will happen every time the aircraft encounters turbulence. Is this really the case? As we will see in Chapter 9, turbulence may be uncomfortable, but it is not dangerous. The following questions may help to challenge inaccurate thinking about turbulence:

- What is actually true about turbulence? (It may be uncomfortable and make me feel unsafe.)
- What facts might I be forgetting or ignoring? (Turbulence does not damage the aircraft; the aircraft is far stronger than required to cope with turbulence; aircraft wings are designed to flex to make turbulence more comfortable – they cannot snap or fall off; the captain usually knows when there is turbulence and will switch the seat-belt sign on.)
- What is *not* true about turbulence? (It is dangerous; the pilots lose control of the aircraft; the aircraft will fall from the sky.)
- What's the worst thing that can happen? (The aircraft shakes for a while; I have to stay in my seat for a period of time; the cabin crew can't serve me hot drinks; I will feel uncomfortable; I will feel anxious.)
- How can I handle my response to turbulence? (I can practise controlled breathing and relaxation techniques to reduce my anxiety; I can distract myself from obsessing about turbulence by reading this book or a magazine, talking to other passengers, listening to my iPod; I can follow the instructions from the captain and remain in my seat with the seat belt fastened until the turbulence has passed.)

Go over each of your worries about flying, one by one. When you come across a misconception, encourage realistic thoughts by asking yourself:

- Are my assumptions true or are my nervous feelings leading me to expect the worst?
- Am I using any thinking errors? (Go back to the list of thinking errors in Chapter 5 and see if you can link any of these to your anxious thoughts.)
- Do I have evidence for my thought?
- Where is the information that will tell me how accurate my thinking is? (Hopefully in this book, but if not, is there anywhere else I can gather more information to challenge my worry?)
- What is a more helpful/realistic way of thinking?

Use the preceding example of turbulence as a model and ask the same questions for each of your anxious thoughts in turn. You may find it a challenge at first to generate alternative explanations for irrational thoughts because you are so used to your negative automatic thoughts! Think about the accurate information with which to replace the thought. Make a grid like the one below, listing your anxious and irrational thoughts and adding helpful alternatives with which to replace them.

| Anxious thoughts | Helpful thoughts |
|---|---|
| Turbulence is dangerous. | |
| Flying is not safe. | |
| I won't be able to get out of the plane – I am stuck. | |
| Something awful is going to happen to me. | |
| I don't feel good – there must be something wrong. | |

Ask yourself the question: 'How come others on this flight are not affected in the same way as me?'

You can use this book and ask other people's views to check whether your assumptions are true. Below is a list of common examples of thoughts that make people feel afraid. It is the same list that you encountered in the table above, but this time we have included alternative thoughts to give examples of how you can challenge worry.

Anxious thought: *'Flying is not safe'*

Flying is far safer than any other form of transportation. What you are really saying is that you feel vulnerable when travelling by air, which is different from the broad assumption that flying is inherently unsafe.

> Alternative thought: *'Hundreds of thousands of people fly every day and land safely at their destinations. The statistics suggest that I am actually safer in the air than travelling by car, boat or train. The pilots have extensive flying training and the aircraft is serviced on a regular basis to ensure technical equipment works properly. While it is true that there is risk involved in everything that we do, I can minimize injury or accidents by following the safety announcements on board the aircraft.'*

> Anxious thought: *'I won't be able to get out of the plane – I am stuck!'*

It is true that you won't be able to get out of the aircraft; the aircraft doors cannot be opened in flight. What you really mean is that you are afraid of not being able to keep calm and relaxed in the confined space of the aircraft cabin. You are fearful of the thought of becoming panicky in front of other people as this could cause feelings of shame and embarrassment. In spite of anything you may be imagining, aircraft doors are built so that they cannot be opened in flight (the system which controls the air in the cabin means there is a lot of pressure keeping the door shut – no human could open it until after landing, when the pressure inside and out becomes the same again).

> Alternative thought: *'Once the seat-belt signs have been switched on I can move around the cabin. This will make the space seem bigger as I will have more room than the immediate area around my seat. When I focus on the need to get out of the cabin my anxiety only gets worse. I feel nervous because the door is securely locked.'*

> Anxious thought: *'Something awful is going to happen to me'*

What do you know or what can you see, hear or touch that makes you think your anxious thoughts might be correct? What do you know or what can you see, hear or touch that might help you change that thought?

> Alternative thought: *'While there is no guarantee that everything will go smoothly, it is equally possible that my plans will turn out perfectly fine. My catastrophizing thoughts almost never come true. I waste a lot of time and energy thinking about what could go wrong when in reality nothing bad ever happens. It is my thoughts that are the 'bad' thing, not the risk of them becoming true. By focusing on the many things that are likely to turn out fine, I am more likely to feel comfortable and calm during the flight.'*

> Anxious thought: *'I feel tense and nervous – something is wrong'*

You think something catastrophic will happen because you feel tense and nervous. You are acting upon your feelings and letting these control your understanding of the environment.

> Alternative thought: *'Just because I feel tense and nervous does not necessarily mean that something will go wrong during the flight. I need to stop paying attention to every step of the journey as it is easy to become fixated on minor details. Besides, since I am not a pilot, my efforts will have little or no bearing on flying safety. I can, however, control the urge to keep watch on everything around me. I can focus on the in-flight entertainment, read my book, and listen to music or think about a pleasant experience such as my friend's wedding last month. This will distract me and help reduce the feelings of nervousness and tension.'*

Once you have identified a worrying thought and constructed a more realistic version, the final stage is to practise your new way of thinking. You may find that you have become so good at anxious thinking that changing your assumptions about flying is quite hard to start with. You may need to practise alternative thinking more than once before you notice any changes to your flying experience. Keep a list of these thoughts so that you can read them through in situations that you feel may give rise to greater anxiety (e.g. when waiting in the departure lounge to board the aircraft). What you should tell yourself is that feeling a bit nervous when flying is normal – but this is all there is to it!

You can continue to worry about everything that could possibly go wrong but this will make your anxiety worse. Instead, you can, and should, decide to focus on making the journey as pleasurable and enjoyable as possible. You can use the extensive checklists in Chapter 10 to help you prepare for a more comfortable and relaxed flight. When you feel tense and anxious, say to yourself:

*'Just because I feel worried doesn't mean that something bad will happen. My worry is self-made and does not necessarily reflect what will happen. I can distract myself by reading my book, eating the in-flight meal, listening to music or watching a comedy on the in-flight entertainment system. I can talk to people around me to make the flight interesting and comfortable. I can cope with the flight – I just need to trust my abilities to manage my anxiety. I can do this!'*

## Redirecting your thoughts

Another approach to managing anxious thoughts is to redirect your attention to something else. If you have found it difficult to challenge your thoughts in the way we have just described, you may find that the techniques we describe here to enable you to redirect your thoughts can help. When we are scared of a situation, our minds tend to attach unhelpful meanings to aspects of ourselves ('I can't cope', 'I am going to faint', 'I will have a panic attack'), the world around us ('turbulence is dangerous', 'what if the engines stop working?') and to other people ('the crew may think I am weird', 'other passengers are looking at me'). We also tend to over-focus on particular aspects of these unhelpful meanings, which can often make the anxiety worse.

Carlos, aged 34, was flying to Moscow for a business meeting. He had not travelled by air for the past two years. The last time Carlos flew, he experienced a panic attack while on board the aircraft. During the entire journey, Carlos kept checking his body for physical signs of panic (*over-focusing*). He directed his attention towards his breathing ('Is my breathing OK?'), his hands ('I am sure my hands are trembling'), his body temperature ('I feel hot') and the pace of his heartbeat ('I need to check my pulse again to ensure the pace of my heartbeats are normal. Is my heart beating too fast?') (*physical symptoms*). The intense focus on bodily symptoms led Carlos to think there was something wrong with him (*interpretation*). He muttered to himself, 'I am going to have a panic attack' (*unhelpful meanings attached to his thoughts*). He felt increasingly uncomfortable and anxious during the entire journey.

You can develop the ability to redirect your attention towards other features of your experience, which can help improve your mood and reduce anxiety. Carlos, for example, may have benefited from directing his attention away from bodily sensations. Rather than thinking about his physical wellbeing, he could have focused his attention towards the external environment (talking to a fellow passenger or watching the crew when they serve drinks) and what he could be doing (listening to his iPod, reading a book, preparing his business meeting, relaxing).

Redirecting your attention can be particularly useful in situations that trigger anxiety. It can help you counterbalance the tendency to focus on threats when you feel anxious. The point of shifting your attention is not to reduce your overall concentration, but to focus harder on different areas of your immediate environment. When you pay too much attention to anxiety-provoking sensations and images, your ability to process information around you is limited. Carlos, for example, could not recall the pleasant manner of the crew or the smoothness of the pilots' take-off and landing. Intentionally directing your attention away from anxious threats does not mean suppressing your thoughts. Instead, you can master choosing what you pay attention to when your anxiety is triggered.

If Carlos had not focused so much on bodily sensations during the flight, the intensity of his anxiety would gradually have decreased. As a consequence, he may have felt more comfortable and been better able to appreciate other aspects of his journey.

Anxious thoughts can make you feel distressed and overwhelmed. They are often characterized by uncertainty and tend to give rise to a number of 'what if ...' questions. Some people say that anxious thoughts are similar to a 'stuck record'; it feels as if the same words are being repeated over and over again in their minds. This is an ideal time to practise distraction techniques. By concentrating on something else you can stop paying attention to your anxious thoughts, which will allow you to feel more comfortable and relaxed. Take a look at the information below, as this will help you identify the thoughts to look out for and when to practise distractions.

**Stop & Think**

Try to identify the distractions most likely to work for you. Plan to use your individual distraction technique next time you take a flight. Please note that certain distractions can inadvertently add pressure. For example, if you were planning to get work done on board the aircraft as a distraction, you may feel more stressed if you fail to complete the planned workload. Therefore, it is important that you choose an easily achievable task and don't over-plan for your journey.

## Concentration exercises

Worry is a natural way of anticipating risk and keeps us safe from catastrophe and danger. It is an automatic skill that is activated when we feel unsafe. When our perception of risk is exaggerated, we are also likely to feel unsafe and hence we start to worry in order to protect ourselves from the imagined fear. This is why anxious thoughts about flying can be intense and persistent. The challenge here is to let go of your worry because it makes the anxiety worse. The following concentration techniques will help you to stop the flow of anxious thoughts, reduce your distress and make you feel more calm and relaxed. As you begin to practise concentrating on a task in hand, try to implement the techniques in situations you regard as less threatening. Once you develop your ability to direct your attention away from the source of your fear, you can move on to use the techniques during more challenging situations.

### Listening to the lyrics of a song

Select a song that you like and play it on your laptop, CD, iPod or cassette player. Concentrate on the lyrics of the song for about two minutes. Turn the playing device off and summarize the lyrics of the song out loud. Note how much of your attention is directed towards the task of listening to the song, yourself and the environment around you. You can use percentages to measure the focus of your attention, as in the following example:

| Concentrating on task | Yourself | The environment |
|---|---|---|
| 40% | 30% | 30% |

Carry out the exercise again, but choose a different song. Try to deliberately distract yourself on this occasion by focusing on your thoughts and sensations before you redirect your concentration towards the lyrics of the song. Summarize the lyrics again and note how you divided your attention between your thoughts, sensations and the task of listening to the song (in percentage terms, as shown above).

Repeat the listening activities until you become adept at redirecting your attention to the task of listening to the words of the song after deliberate distraction through focusing on yourself. This will help to develop your ability to control where and when you focus your attention.

### Paying attention to your surroundings

This exercise asks you to pay attention to the entirety of your surroundings: what you can see, feel, hear and smell. The value of this is to help you shift your focus from your worry towards the more pleasant and positive aspects of your surroundings. You can use almost any situation to practise shifting your attention towards the outside world. This includes walking to your local food store, a trip in the park, attending a social event, visiting a museum, travelling to work or making a special meal for supper. Here is a pre-flight exercise that can help you shift your attention away from anxious thoughts about flying. It will allow you to feel more in control of your thoughts and strengthen the belief that you can cope with your flying anxiety.

- Focus your attention for about six minutes on the different aspects of your surroundings.
- First, focus your attention mainly on what you can see (colours, objects, and people).
- After about one minute begin to shift your attention towards what you can hear – the various noises around you.
- Then shift your attention to concentrate on smells before you redirect the focus towards your feelings.
- Keep moving your attention to these different sensations. Try to vary the order of your attention to the individual sensations as this will help develop your skills for controlling your attention. Notice how you feel much more relaxed once you direct your attention away from yourself.

- Next, try to integrate your attention to include all aspects of your surroundings. Use percentages to measure the degree to which you are paying attention to the different aspects of the environment (what you can see, feel, hear and smell).

When seated in the aircraft cabin, you can use attention retraining to help prevent yourself from engaging with the stream of worry that accompanies flying anxiety. While preparing for a flight or even during a flight, you are probably focusing your attention towards yourself and fail to perceive other aspects around you. This means that you are likely to miss out on the positive and interesting parts of the journey. With practice you can train yourself to tune into the world around you, even during threatening situations. Below is a list of tasks you can attend to during the flight:

- Focus on what you can hear, smell and see on board the aircraft.
- Read your book/magazine and try to summarize each page before you progress to the next one.
- Listen to music and memorize the words of the song.

## Changing your behaviour

We now turn our attention towards techniques which focus on changing behaviours that may be maintaining your fear of flying. When driven by fear, people often behave in ways that are different from their usual habits of responding. They may not even be conscious of their actions during the heat of an anxious moment. Paul, for example, used to clench his body so hard during take-off and landing that he felt physically ill after a flight. He only became aware of this habit after a colleague brought it to his attention during a business trip abroad. Up until then, Paul had not realized what he was doing, and neither was he aware of the ill effects of the clenching on his physical health.

There are times when we only become aware of our behaviour after the situation has occurred – when the fear has settled down. This can sometimes lead us to feel as if we have no choice over our actions: 'I can't help it'. Clare had a habit of squeezing the arm rest very tightly during a flight. She knew that her action was not going to make a difference to the course of the flight; by holding on tightly she was not going to stop or prevent aircraft turbulence. Still, she found it difficult to let go because it made her feel a little bit better. However, Clare's behaviour actually made her feel more tense, anxious and uncomfortable. Although her actions were driven by the understandable goal to reduce her fear of turbulence, she ended up reinforcing the belief that she needed to 'hold on tightly', which was a major part of her problem (feeling unsafe when flying). The 'clenching behaviour' can be reduced by practising the relaxation/breathing techniques in Chapter 8. This will allow you to release the physical tension that accompanies flying anxiety and make you feel calm and relaxed.

There are other times when we are aware of those habits that relate to fear but find it difficult to change them. How many times, for example, have you attempted to put off dealing with a problem? Unfortunately, this can make things worse in the long term and can be counterproductive. Consider a time when you waited to take action until the last minute. This might have involved preparing for a business meeting, revising for an exam, or even telling a friend that you could not make her birthday party. It may have saved you some discomfort (and perhaps even boredom!) in the short term but it is also likely that the undone task played on your mind for quite some time. This is not to mention the increase in stress level you may have endured when discovering that the problem had escalated out of control because you failed to deal with it in time.

One of the most common ways of reducing fear of flying is to avoid flying. This is unhelpful because it prevents you from confronting your fear and is likely to make your flying anxiety worse. We now introduce techniques to help you reduce avoidance.

## Dealing with avoidance

Avoidance, more than any other behaviour, will maintain worry, fear and anxiety about air travel. This section is designed to help you to give up avoidance. Facing what you fear is the most important aspect of overcoming it. Through avoidance, a person may never get the chance to discover whether or not that fear is real, and never have the opportunity to deal with that fear and overcome it. Before you go on to develop the skills to help you face your fear, it is advisable that you first learn how to deal with the unpleasant bodily sensations of anxiety and your worrying thoughts.

Tackling your fear one step at a time is known as graded practice. Although the notion of facing your fear of flying might seem alarming, you can learn to do it gradually, so that you never feel too afraid all at once. You can start by attempting something that you are less fearful of and then move on to more challenging situations at your own pace. It's a little bit like climbing a hill that gradually gets steeper as you approach the top. During your climb you are likely to gain confidence about your trekking skills, the surroundings and your ability to get to the top. By learning to face your fear one step at a time, you are gradually building up your confidence and motivation to cope with flying anxiety.

There are three steps in graded practice:

1  Identify your fear(s) and set the target(s).
2  Grade the task(s) from less fearful to most fearful.
3  Keep practising each of the tasks in the list until you are ready to move to the next step.

Before you are in a position to set a target, it is important that you describe your fear in detail. You might say that you are afraid of flying but this can mean quite different things for different people. The following questions may help you to think about your own fear:

- What is it about air travel that scares you the most (turbulence, heights, confined spaces, lack of control, fear of death, security, etc.)?
- Are there any other situations that resemble your fear (turbulence – rides on a fairground; heights – taking the lift to the top floor of a high building; confined spaces – being in a crowded place; other people – attending a large party/social gathering, etc.)?
- Is there a point when you notice an increase in your anxiety level (booking the air ticket; the lead-up period to the journey; travelling to the airport; seeing other aircraft; check-in; security; sitting in the airport lounge; during boarding; during take-off; when there is turbulence; during the landing; or all of the situations mentioned)?
- Does it make a difference what airline you fly with, the duration of the flight or the size of the aircraft?
- Does it make a difference if you are travelling with someone, the characteristics and behaviours of the person(s) travelling with you?
- Does it make a difference if airline staff act in a warm, professional and friendly manner?
- Does it make a difference if the weather forecast is good?
- Does it make a difference if the ability to complete the journey is of high importance to your relationships, career or wellbeing?
- Is there anything else that makes you more or less anxious about a particular flight (perhaps where you sit on the aircraft or the reason for travelling)?

When you have asked yourself these questions, you can explore your fear in more detail. You might discover that your fear of flying is only triggered on long-haul journeys and that you can tolerate shorter flights. You may find that you do not like sitting towards the back of the aircraft but you feel reasonably comfortable when sitting in the middle or at the front, or that you feel less anxious when you travel with a larger airline than with smaller aviation companies. Make a note of your fear, for example:

**My fear 1**
*Fear of long-haul journeys that gets worse if I am sitting towards the very back of the aircraft and travelling with a smaller airline company.*

You may have more than one specific fear about flying. You can do this exercise for each aspect of flying that you fear:

**My fear 2**
*Fear of travelling alone that gets worse if the airport is crowded with people and there is a long queue at security.*

The next step is to arrange your fears in order of difficulty, for example:

**Most difficult**
*1) Travelling on a long-haul journey*
*2) Sitting towards the back of the aircraft*
*3) Travelling with a small aviation company*

**Least difficult**
*4) Travelling alone*
*5) Being in a crowded place*
*6) Queuing up for security.*

When you have your targets ranked according to difficulty, select the easiest one to start with. At this stage, you should only tackle one at a time. If you are afraid of both turbulence and travelling on long-haul journeys, you may find that you are able to tackle both at the same time. Remember that each challenge provides an opportunity to use the coping skills outlined in this and the next chapter (challenging anxious thoughts and redirecting your attention, controlled breathing and relaxation).

You now need to plan a series of small, specific tasks of increasing difficulty. The first task has to be achievable, so it may be worth asking yourself: Which one of these targets would I definitely be able to carry out? Your graded practice may look something like this:

**Target 1** (least difficult): Fear of travelling alone that gets worse if the airport is crowded and there is a long queue at security.

1 Queuing up and going through security by myself when I am travelling with my husband on a short-haul flight to Glasgow.
2 Going to the shops on a Saturday when it is busy to get used to being in a crowd. Entering the airport terminal by myself when travelling with my husband to Glasgow.
3 Travelling by myself on a short-haul journey to Amsterdam. My sister will pick me up from the terminal when I arrive.

*Target 2* (moderately difficult): Fear of travelling with smaller airline companies that gets worse if I am sitting towards the back of the aircraft.

4 Booking a charter flight with a smaller airline company for my next holiday.
5 On the return journey I could try and ask for a seat towards the back of the aircraft for my husband and me.

*Target 3* (most difficult): Fear of travelling on longer flights.

6 Travelling on a medium-distance flight to Cyprus to visit relatives.
7 Try and book a long-haul flight to New York next year.

Before you introduce your plan to overcome avoidance, it is important that you think about what you want to be able to do, as this can have a positive effect on your motivation. It is worth noting that your list of graded practice is likely to be specific to your fear and your personal needs, wants and desires. A second consideration is to try and make your goals as realistic as possible, so as to ensure they are achievable. You may want to think about what type of resources to build into your graded practice (e.g. a partner who flies for work, finances to fund flying experiences, relatives to go and visit, friends to go on holiday with, etc.). If you find that a task is too difficult, don't give up or feel that you have failed. Instead, look for ways to make the task easier, perhaps by breaking it into smaller steps.

Remember to plan in advance what techniques you are going to use to approach each step of your graded practice. You can use the techniques described in this book, such as challenging your anxious thoughts and attention retraining, as well as breathing and relaxation techniques. Expect some setbacks as these are normally a part of the road to recovery. You may feel anxious, which is only natural as you are learning to manage your anxiety instead of avoiding it. Ensure that you reward yourself for your efforts and achievements. You deserve praise for your bravery and persistent fight to overcome your fear!

As we have seen, you can learn to overcome your fear of flying by learning to challenge distressing thoughts and changing unhelpful behaviours. The techniques presented in this chapter are based on cognitive behavioural therapy. The aim is to teach you effective skills for managing your flying anxiety. Cognitive behavioural therapy, however, is not a miraculous 'quick fix' approach that can 'cure' you of all your problems. Rather, it is a skills-based approach that gradually allows you to build up your confidence and repertoire of techniques for dealing with flying anxiety. As you continue to practise the techniques described in this book, you will notice a steady progression over time that empowers you to manage your fear.

The next chapter focuses on the physical symptoms of your anxiety. It is important that you learn how to deal with bodily distress, as this can make your fear of flying worse. Controlled breathing and relaxation techniques are easy to apply and will help you feel calm and comfortable when you are taking a flight.

# 8

# Learning how to relax

Learning relaxation skills is vital for treating a fear of flying because it helps you to manage the bodily symptoms we described in Chapter 4. These skills will help you build a sense of control over these symptoms and enable you to feel more confident. They will also help you to reinforce the belief that you can cope with difficult situations. Learning how to control bodily symptoms of anxiety is a skill that needs be practised frequently before you can expect lasting benefits and mastery. It is a bit like learning to drive a car; you need to keep practising until you are able to coordinate the many skills required to operate the vehicle without consciously thinking about them. It can be difficult at first, especially if you try to apply relaxation skills during a challenging situation. It is therefore important to practise first in settings where you feel comfortable.

This chapter presents a number of relaxation techniques that will help to reduce your anxiety, stress and tension. We first focus on relaxed, controlled ways of breathing, before moving on to teach you how to release physical tension and relax your body and mind. These are important skills that can help you feel calmer and more comfortable when you are faced with a challenging task or distressing situation. Once you have learnt practical skills for reducing the bodily signs of anxiety, you will be in a much better frame of mind to tackle the unpleasant thoughts and behavioural elements that maintain your flying anxiety.

Although the physical experience of fear and anxiety is normal, it can cause high levels of discomfort if the reaction is misinterpreted or excessive. If your bodily reactions are extreme, the experience can be frightening and distressing enough to give rise to two challenges: the unpleasant effects of anxiety coupled with a fear of experiencing these symptoms. They have the further effect of reinforcing one another. Anticipation of physical discomfort, nausea, sweating, breathing difficulties or tightening in the chest, to name a few, can then produce the stress that reinforces these bodily sensations. Table 8.1 gives examples of the many ways in which symptoms of physical discomfort can be misinterpreted.

**Table 8.1 Misinterpretation of symptoms of physical discomfort**

| Bodily changes | What is happening | Misinterpretations |
|---|---|---|
| Shallow, rapid breathing | Hyperventilation – you are using only the upper parts of the lungs and this results in the inhalation of too much oxygen | 'I can't breathe. I am suffocating' |
| Muscle tightening in the chest area, headaches | Tension – muscular tension causes uncomfortable sensations such as headaches, tightness in chest area, pains, etc. | 'This is a heart attack I am having a stroke' |
| Nausea and dizziness | When the oxygen level in your body rises (hyperventilation), the relative carbon dioxide level falls below normal. This imbalance causes unpleasant symptoms including nausea and light-headedness | 'I will collapse. I will faint. I will make a fool of myself' |
| Sweating, trembling, hot and flushed | Bodily temperature rises because of physical exertion brought on by hyperventilation and muscular tension | 'I can't cope. I am weak' |

There is a range of techniques that can help you to modify the bodily responses associated with fear of flying. We have found relaxed and controlled breathing and applied relaxation to be particularly effective ways of producing physical relief. These are widely recognized methods for coping with bodily sensations during anxiety attacks. They are designed to tackle hyperventilation (over-breathing) and muscle tension respectively. As we demonstrated in Table 8.1, rapid shallow breathing and muscular tension are thought to maintain and reinforce many of the unpleasant sensations associated with your fear of flying. It therefore makes sense to deal with each of these in turn. You may already be familiar with breathing exercises and healthy ways of resting, especially if you practise yoga, meditation or have completed a course in relaxation skills. If this is the case, the techniques described below can be used to build on existing skills to enhance your repertoire for relaxation.

## Relaxed, controlled breathing

We tend to over-breathe whenever we are tense or when we are exercising. This is a mild form of hyperventilation that increases blood circulation so that our muscles can be primed to react during activity. We notice that our heart rate increases, our breathing becomes more irregular and muscles may tense up slightly. Rapid breathing is not problematic in the short term. It is a perfectly healthy response to ensure we can sustain exercise, whether working out in the gym, running a marathon or speeding towards the office to make the morning meeting. It is also a normal response to stress and anxiety.

**Stop & Think**

Think about the last time you exercised. This might involve attending a fitness class at your local gym, physical activity with your children in the garden or running to catch a bus. What happened to your breathing (slower, faster, rapid, shallow)? Did you notice any bodily changes (heavier breathing, increased body temperature, muscle aches especially in the leg area, heart palpitations)? How did you control these physical sensations (slowed down the pace, regular rest periods, deep breathing techniques)? What happened to your breathing once you stopped exercising or slowed the pace down? Did you continue to over-breathe or did you find that the pace of your breathing naturally slowed down?

Continued rapid breathing can cause intense physical discomfort, which can be quite frightening. Imagine that you are sitting in the airport terminal feeling anxious about your flight. Your breathing is getting heavier; you become hot and flushed. You may be thinking, 'What is happening to me?' and 'I am never going to get through the flight.' There are two things happening to your mind and body here: your initial fear of flying has caused over-breathing, which triggers off a range of physical sensations that can be quite uncomfortable. These have led you to develop a second fear, 'I won't be able to control myself.'

Although it is common to worry about losing control, it is very unlikely that you will. It may feel as if the pain may never end and you may worry that you won't be able to restore your breathing to a healthy state. This is a common response to continuous over-breathing. Being able to correct over-breathing is a very powerful way of reducing these unpleasant physical sensations. You can easily learn to correct over-breathing by developing the habit of 'correct' breathing. Although breathing comes naturally and we all do it without even thinking, there is a tendency to lose our normal ways of breathing when we are afraid, such as of flying. The breathing technique that follows will help you to develop the ability to control symptoms of over-breathing. You can apply the technique in almost any situation: while sitting in the airport lounge, queuing up with fellow passengers to board the flight or when seated on board the aircraft.

The overall goal of this breathing technique is to learn a way to relax through breathing. It involves learning to take gentle, even breaths that fill your lungs completely and then to exhale slowly and steadily. You should start by practising this technique in a comfortable situation when you are not too stressed or anxious. Each exercise should last for about ten minutes and you should ideally practise twice a day if you can: once in the morning and once in the evening. Find a quiet place that is free from distractions and noise. This could be in your office, at home, in the garden or even at your local gym. When you first start practising, you may want to ensure you are alone, as it is easy to lose focus when other people are around to distract you. You are also more likely to feel self-conscious if your partner or friend is watching when you practise relaxing and controlled breathing.

- Before you start, it is important that you feel comfortable and able to relax. You can practise controlled breathing in a seated position with your hands relaxed on either side of your body, or with your back flat on the ground in a lying position. If you practise in a lying position, you may find it more comfortable to support your back by placing a pillow or cushion underneath your knees.
- Loosen any tight clothing and take off your shoes if you can.
- Let your shoulder blades sink down your back, and lean slightly towards the back of the chair (or the ground if you are lying down) to support your back. Close your eyes.
- Start by taking a deep breath in through your nose and exhaling slowly through your mouth. Continue to breathe in through your nose and out through your mouth about five more times.
- Try to make each inhalation and exhalation of the same duration. When you inhale, count slowly from 1 through to 4. Do the same when you exhale, so that you are breathing evenly in a slow and focused manner. Notice how your breathing slows down.

- Feel the way your lungs gradually expand on every in breath. As you breathe out you are emptying your lungs. Your body feels relaxed. Continue to breathe slowly ... in through your nose and out through your mouth.
- Place your right hand on your tummy and let it rest lightly on top of your navel. As you breathe in through your nose, feel the way your tummy rises. As you breathe out through your mouth, your hand is sinking further and further down towards the middle part of your body until your tummy feels completely flat.
- Your heartbeat is slowing down. Your arms and legs are relaxed. Continue to count slowly from 1 to 4 on each inhalation and then again for each exhalation.
- On each out breath, imagine that you are pushing the tension out of your lungs. Let it flow through your mouth and out into the wider world. You are getting rid of all the tension, stress and worry.
- Let go of all bodily tension whatsoever. Continue to breathe deeply five more times ... in through your nose and out through your mouth. Feel the quietness and peacefulness around you.
- Slowly open your eyes. Continue to breathe gently and evenly in through your nose and out through your mouth. Gently move your legs and arms. If you are in a seated position, raise your arms and stretch the whole of your body upwards. If you are lying down, flex your arms and legs downwards and gently move back up into a seated position.

You may find it a challenge to practise controlled breathing at first. You may feel as if you are not getting enough air or that the pace of your breathing seems unnaturally slow. This is a normal reaction when you practise a new routine. If you find it difficult to read the instructions while carrying out the breathing routine (most of us do!), you may benefit from recording the instructions with lots of pauses and playing them back the first few times you practise. As your skill improves and you learn to relax quickly, you will find it easier to switch to correct breathing whenever you feel anxious. You may want to progress to more distracting situations with your eyes open – such as, for example, getting the kids off to school! This will improve your skills and help you to control your breathing while taking a flight abroad. The technique is simple and can be used at any stage of your flying experience. It is easy to apply and will help to reduce tension, anxiety and stress.

# Releasing physical tension

Once you have learnt the skill of relaxing your muscles, your mind and body will automatically feel calmer. It is almost impossible for the mind to be tense when the body is relaxed. The ability to relax is not always something that comes easily; it is a skill that needs to be learnt gradually and practised regularly.

As we have seen, anxiety is different for each of us. We may not have the same bodily symptoms; each of us has our own independent anxious thoughts and each of us behaves differently when under stress. It is therefore important that you find a relaxation technique that works for you. This is best done by regular practice before taking a flight, so that you get used to doing it and gain confidence in its benefits. The aim is to learn relaxation techniques in advance so that you are in a better position to manage your anxiety on your day of travel.

How quickly it is possible to reduce the physical symptoms of anxiety will vary from one person to another. It will depend upon the severity of your anxiety, your ability to relax during periods of stress and the nature of the muscle tensions involved. Nevertheless, relaxation methods have a very good chance of success if you practise them regularly and take them seriously.

## Monitoring progress

Before you begin to practise relaxation skills, spend a minute or two on identifying the intensity of your stress and anxiety levels. This can be done by asking yourself: How tense/stressed/anxious do I feel right now? Use a scale from 1 (low) to 10 (high) to rate the degree of tenseness/stress/anxiety:

| How tense, stressed and/ or anxious do I feel? | Before relaxation 1 (low) to 10 (high) | After relaxation 1 (low) to 10 (high) |
|---|---|---|
| Tense | | |
| Stressed | | |
| Anxious | | |

Work through the first of the exercises provided below. Once you have finished the exercise, take a further measure of your anxiety. Compare the two sets of scores and see whether you feel less tense/anxious/ stressed (or if there is no change) after completing the relaxation sequence. Repeat this procedure for each exercise. You need to know if the relaxation procedure works for you, though there may be some minor variation from day to day.

## Progressive muscular relaxation

The first exercise will help you to distinguish between tensed and relaxed muscles. This will help you to identify when you are tense so that you can learn to relax your muscles. Muscular tension can occur automatically as a reaction to uncomfortable thoughts and worry. We are not always conscious of physical tension and it is therefore not uncommon for people to experience prolonged periods of muscular strain. This exercise will increase your awareness of bodily tension and can therefore act as a cue, letting you know when it may be beneficial to apply relaxation techniques to help let go of muscular strain. The sequence is quite simple and takes you through all parts of your body. This exercise is best done in a lying position, but if this is difficult, sitting in a chair can work equally well. Once you are confident with the technique, you should practise it when sitting as this is the position you will be in while flying. You can use the controlled breathing techniques in the previous exercise to enhance relaxation and calmness. Remember to make a note of how anxious/stressed you are before starting the exercise.

The basic movements which you can use for each part of your body are as follows; tense the muscles as much as you can (within reason) and concentrate on feeling the strain within your body. Hold the tension for about five seconds and then release your muscles. Relax the muscle for 15 seconds and note the difference between the tense and relaxed state of your muscle. Use this basic technique on each muscle group in turn. Remember to breathe gently and evenly throughout the exercise.

- **Hands**. Clench your left hand and make a tight fist. Then relax your left hand – let it sink towards the ground. Do the same with your right hand.
- **Arms**. Tense your whole arm. Imagine that you are holding a set of weights in your hand. Bring the bottom half of your arm upwards as this will make it easier to flex your arm. Relax for 15 seconds. Repeat the process for your right arm.
- **Face**. Tense your eyebrows by frowning, then your forehead and jaws. Relax for 15 seconds and repeat.
- **Neck and shoulders**. Let your chin drop down towards your chest. Squeeze your shoulders up towards your neck as hard as you can.

Hold for 15 seconds and then relax. Repeat the process once more. As your shoulders release, feel your shoulder blades slide gently down your back towards your waist.

- **Abdomen.** Tighten the muscles in your stomach by pulling them in and up. Hold for five seconds and then relax for 15 seconds. Repeat the tensing and relax again.
- **Thighs.** Relax your upper body. Tighten your thigh muscles by squeezing your buttocks and thighs together. Relax for 15 seconds, then repeat the process.
- **Legs.** Bend your feet downwards so that your toes are pointing towards the floor. There should be a tightening sensation in the back of your leg muscles. Relax for 15 seconds. Then bend your feet the other way so that your toes are pointing upwards. You should feel a light tension in the front part of your legs. Relax.
- **The whole of your body.** Tense all of the above body parts at once. You should feel a tension in your hands, face area, neck and shoulders, abdomen, thighs and legs. Relax for 15 seconds and then repeat this process once more.

Take care not to over-tense muscles, as this can cause discomfort or even injury to your body. Remember to breathe slowly and regularly between each part of the exercise. When you have finished the sequence, spend a minute or two thinking about something pleasant – for example, a relaxing walk along the seafront or eating a piece of your favourite chocolate cake. This will allow a gentle transition back into your normal environment. Before you stand up straight, gently stretch and move your arms and legs, avoiding sudden or jerky movements.

When you are ready, take your time standing up. If you still feel tense at the end of the exercise, try and go through the sequence once more. Remember, it takes time to learn how to relax. Give yourself a chance and do not expect to succeed too soon.

Once you have mastered this muscle-relaxing exercise, you can shorten it by missing out the tensing stage. Go through the routine systematically, focusing on each of the muscle groups for 15 to 20 seconds at a time. You can adapt the exercise so that you are able to apply the relaxation procedure while at work, at home, during train journeys or anywhere else you can think of.

The space on board an aircraft is restricted and can often be quite noisy. If you are used to practising relaxation skills only in a 'heavenly calm sanctuary', you may be put off by the external distractions in the aircraft cabin. Learning to relax in a range of different environments is important, because this is what you need for coping in the real world.

You can use relaxation skills the night before you travel, on the bus or train journey to the airport, in the airport lounge and when you are seated on board the aircraft.

## Deep relaxation

The next exercise is a form of distraction and is designed to help you to learn to calm yourself down. You may need to practise the sequence a number of times. It will help you to use a mental image to relax yourself on board the aircraft. Before you start the exercise, remember to note your anxiety/tension level and compare it at the end. For this exercise, you will need to imagine a soothing, restful situation. The mental image will help you relax even more effectively. Here are some suggestions to help you get started:

- a particular place you have visited that you associate with peacefulness and calmness, for example a deserted beach, your holiday home, your garden, the views from the top of a mountain, watching the rain drum against your window or the scenery during a visit to the countryside;
- a poem, song lyric, word or memorable phrase that brings positive images to your mind;
- a pleasant object or person or a movie or picture that you particularly like.

When you have decided what mental image you will use, follow the instructions below. Again, it may be useful to record these including lots of pauses and to play the recording back to guide your first few practice sessions.

- Sit in a comfortable position with your eyes closed.
- Start by focusing on your breathing – listen to the sounds of your breaths.
- When you inhale, fill your lungs completely; exhale by slowly letting go of the air. Slow your breathing down.
- As you continue to breathe, focus on your mental image – the things that you can see, hear and smell. Simply let go of all tension and allow your mind and body to relax.
- Feel your body growing heavier and heavier. Stay with the image and continue to breathe naturally and steadily. Keep the exercise going for 15 to 20 minutes.
- When you have finished, open your eyes and sit in the same position for a minute or two. Slowly move your limbs and prepare yourself to stand up.

## Regular exercise

Another way to become more relaxed is to engage in regular exercise. Exercise helps your body to relieve tension caused by anxiety and stress. There are many different forms of exercise, some of which are 'lighter' than others. They include going for a brisk walk, walking up a set of stairs as opposed to taking the lift/escalator, going to the gym, going for a run, mountain walking, cycling, ballroom dancing and attending a yoga class, to name just a few.

There are several ways to exercise both in the airport terminal and on board the aircraft. Of course, they do not include intense forms of training such as preparing for a marathon! Light forms of physical activity include walking; stretching your body while seated; flexing and moving your feet, ankles, toes, hands, shoulders and wrists while in your aircraft seat; and walking to the toilet or the galley area to enhance the blood circulation in your body. Many in-flight magazines and some in-flight entertainment systems will describe or show you suitable exercise routines.

The following are among the positive effects of regular exercise:

- Exercise can have a positive effect on your mood. Exercise stimulates various brain chemicals, which can leave you feeling happier and more relaxed.
- Exercise delivers blood, oxygen and nutrients to your tissues. In fact, regular exercise helps your entire cardiovascular system work more efficiently.
- Regular exercise can help you fall asleep faster and deepen your sleep.
- Exercise has a positive effect on your health, weight and overall vitality.

You can start exercising by setting yourself small goals such as walking to the shops instead of driving, signing up for gym classes at your local leisure centre, or digging your bicycle out of the garage. While at the airport, you can walk around the shops or carry out gentle stretches when sitting down in the terminal. When the seat-belt signs are off during the flight, don't be afraid to stand up in the aisle to stretch your body or move around the aircraft. This is especially important on longer flights, as sitting in the same position for long periods can be both mentally and physically tiring.

## Applying relaxation techniques

The ability to relax is a skill that can help reduce the bodily symptoms of anxiety. For some people, the anticipation of physical symptoms can be more disturbing than the actual flight itself. In other words, they fear the upsetting experience of the fear. As we have seen in this chapter, controlled breathing and relaxation are an important part of managing your fear of flying that can help reduce physical distress, but they may need to be practised several times before you can expect to discover the effectiveness of their use. We now turn our attention to the technical aspects of flying. The next chapter presents invaluable information that will help you challenge irrational thoughts about flying.

# 9

# Questions fearful flyers ask

This chapter is based on the questions which we have been asked by people who are fearful about flying. Some questions are about how aircraft fly, safety, the weather and so on – the technical things that many passengers, nervous or not, may want to know. We also find that anxious flyers often ask questions that start with 'What if …' We have included some of these as well. Most books on fear of flying start by giving a lot of statistics and technical information about aircraft, flight and flight safety. We have not done this, because the focus of this book is on the way in which our thoughts and behaviour interact to produce fear and on how anxious thoughts and unhelpful behaviours can be addressed. However, we have included this chapter because we want to give you enough information to produce constructive ways of thinking using the skills and techniques explained in this book, particularly in Chapter 7.

You probably will not need to read the whole chapter; in fact, you may not need to read any of it. People have two ways of using information about something that makes them afraid or anxious. For some, information helps them understand what they were worried about and is one of the things that reduces anxiety. For others, information is something they don't want to have and if they are made to read it, they find themselves becoming more anxious. If you find that you do not want to read about it, or even that you are becoming fearful, then skip this chapter.

## Answering your questions

We cannot answer every possible question. We have included some general principles which should help. The reading list at the end of the book should have something that will help if you need more information and most of the books listed will be in your local library.

**Stop & Think**

Before you read the answer to your question, try and think what it is that worries you or makes you want to know that particular answer. What was the *thinking* that made you ask the question? When you have understood the answer, write down a new way of thinking about what was worrying you.

Chapter 7 describes how to challenge your anxious thoughts in detail and you will need to work through the techniques given there to get maximum benefit from creating new ways of thinking. Here is an example of challenging an anxious thought which many people have told us about:

'I wanted to know what causes turbulence and why the aircraft wings flex or "flap" when flying in turbulence, because I thought that bad turbulence could actually make the wings snap off.'

*Turbulence is simply what happens to an aircraft when it flies through air which is rapidly changing direction. If air was visible like water, you would be able to see it like waves on the sea. Pilots have a lot of information which helps them avoid turbulence and they will take extra fuel to fly around it or use another route if they need to. However, sometimes aircraft will fly into turbulence and they are built to be stronger than necessary to do this. The wings flex because this is what they are designed to do; being flexible actually means they are stronger. If I do fly through turbulence, it probably will not last very long. It will be more comfortable if I sit well into my seat with my seat belt not too loose; I'd only get hurt if I stood up and fell over.*

The information given in this chapter will be useful in challenging anxious thoughts that relate to how aircraft fly, safety and the like. We have included some more examples of how to use this information but to make it work best for you, it needs to be done in your own words.

Many people tell us that they often vividly imagine what they think are disasters when they think about flying, and that this makes them anxious. The 'what if ...' questions should help if you find yourself thinking like that. Instead of letting your imagination increase your worries, use it to reduce your anxiety by basing what you imagine will happen on the information in this chapter.

For example:

'I imagine that if I fly, an engine will fail and that will lead to a crash'

*It's very unlikely that an engine will fail. To make absolutely sure that flying is safe, all passenger aircraft have to be able to fly even if an engine fails at the worst possible moment. Pilots are trained to deal with this situation and have to prove that they can do it correctly every six months. If an engine does fail, the pilots will keep the aircraft secure and flying in the right direction. They will land as soon as possible and although I might be delayed getting to where I want to be, I will get there safely.*

Use your imagination to picture a safe flight where even if the engine were to fail, you would land safely.

## General information to think about

Before we move on to answer specific questions, here are some general points about air travel which will be useful to think about when you read some of the other chapters, or are looking for answers we have not given here. These points should help keep your thinking realistic:

- **Aircraft are built with many more working systems than they need.** All aircraft are designed with 'redundant systems' so that if one stops working properly, another takes over. For example, most modern passenger aircraft have three navigation systems, three or four hydraulic systems to move the flying controls or brakes and three sets of instruments. All of these will work independently and if one does stop working properly, another will normally take over automatically.
- **Pilots are always in contact with someone.** In most parts of the world, passenger aircraft only fly on routes in 'controlled airspace'. These are routes through countries or between airports that are designed to ensure that all aircraft are kept safely apart from one another. No aircraft is allowed to fly in controlled airspace without permission from the air traffic controllers who manage that particular area and they must all follow the controllers' instructions. Air traffic controllers have radar systems which identify all the aircraft in the area they are responsible for. This means that the air traffic controllers know about every aircraft in the area, keeping them safely apart and monitoring their progress towards their destination. Aircraft and air traffic controllers use well-maintained radios to talk to each other. If a radio does fail, each aircraft has at least one spare. Even if that were to fail as well, there are procedures to follow which will allow the aircraft to land safely. Many aircraft even have another communication system which works through satellites and can send voice and text messages. The most eventful solution to any communication problem would be using a pair of military aircraft to guide the aircraft with no radio to a safe airport. In the extremely unlikely event that an aircraft's navigation systems develop a fault

or the pilots need assistance, air traffic controllers are highly trained to help. When flying in some parts of the world where immediate contact with air traffic control isn't possible, aircraft follow set routes and are given set times to start and finish these, so as to avoid getting near other aircraft. In such areas, pilots use the radio to talk to other aircraft so that they are all aware of each other.

- **Aircraft have computer systems that constantly monitor their safety**. There are two or three computer systems in all modern passenger aircraft that constantly monitor all the other computer, navigation, electric and hydraulic systems and the engines. If any of these start to work at less than the very highest level of safety, these computers generate messages that tell the pilots or engineers, often before anything noticeable occurs. These systems monitor each other to make sure that they are working correctly.

- **Aircraft manufacturers have to prove the aircraft is safe before it can carry passengers**. The manufacturers must prove that every aircraft can cope with extreme weather conditions and any possible technical fault and that the engines are reliable.

- **Aircraft have several protective systems**. To fly with passengers, modern aircraft have to be fitted with several systems which are designed to protect them. These include:

  ○ many levels of protection to make sure that aircraft do not fly too close to one another. As a first level, pilots are trained to look for other aircraft and to make sure they stay at a safe distance. Even when flying at night or in cloud, air traffic controllers can see every aircraft on their radar displays and will make sure they are safely separated. As an additional protection, all modern aircraft must have collision avoidance systems which make sure that they do not fly too close to one another. Each aircraft has a transmitter that tells air traffic control and other aircraft where it is and what height it is flying at. Aircraft within 40 miles are displayed to the pilots. If any come closer than permitted by a very high level of safety, the system gives an audible warning to the pilots, allowing them to look for the other aircraft and avoid it if necessary. If the aircraft get slightly closer, but well before they are too close, the two transmitters talk to each other and agree a way of avoiding each other. The systems issue these commands to the pilots, who follow them once they have checked it is safe to do so. Typically one aircraft will climb and the other will descend;

  ○ weather radar, which detects most turbulence, storms and heavy showers so that pilots can plan a route around them;

  ○ ground proximity warning systems which stop aircraft flying too close to hills or mountains. These use a combination of a ground detecting radio system and a worldwide database of ground heights. The system knows where the aircraft is and how high the ground is at that point and checks this with the radio system. If the aircraft flies closer to the ground than very high levels of safety demand, the system warns the pilots and they are trained to immediately climb.

- **Cabin crew and pilots have to train and practise for any emergency.** Before flying, cabin crew have to train and pass practical and written exams in first aid, know where all the safety equipment on the aircraft is and how to use it and practise for any possible emergency. Pilots have to train and practise for emergencies that the majority will never even hear of happening throughout their career.

## Technical questions we have been asked

These are the questions we have most often been asked by passengers and fearful flyers. We have included the ones which are most likely to cause anxious thoughts.

### How safe is flying?

We find that this question is often asked by people who are anxious that getting on an aircraft will mean that they are more likely to have a traumatic experience than if they stay at home. In fact, one study showed that the accident rate at home is so high and flying is so safe that a statistician would tell you it is 17 times safer to take a flight than to stay at home! You would have to take a one-way flight with a UK airline every day for 3,500 years to be sure of being involved in a major accident; even then, most passengers would only suffer minor injuries. Most other countries have similar safety records.

There is an enormous number of statistics we could quote to show just how safe flying is. You may already know some of them. Whichever statistics you look at, commercial air travel with a Western airline is one of the safest forms of travel. Problems do happen with any form of transport, but flying is one of the most highly regulated ways to travel, in order to make sure that it is as safe as possible.

As we have stressed throughout this book, there is a difference between understanding that flying is safe and being able to control thoughts that you might be one of the few who are involved in traumatic experiences. We've included a couple of 'headline' statistics here so that you can use them to help create new ways of thinking as you work through the book.

## If flying is safe, why do the cabin crew do a safety demonstration every time?

It is natural to think that airlines insist on safety demonstrations because they expect something to go wrong. It's actually almost the complete opposite: the safety demonstration is done on every flight to make sure that you have all the information you need to be as safe as possible. It's done for the same reasons that cinemas have big emergency exit signs and cruise liners carry out lifeboat drills. No one expects anything to go wrong, but airlines carry safety equipment and give safety demonstrations to give everyone the highest possible level of safety. In the UK and most other countries, the safety demonstration is required by law.

You may also notice that the cabin crew behave differently when they're carrying out the safety demonstration and checking the cabin afterwards. As you came on board, you were probably greeted with a smile and you may have been offered a drink. During the safety demonstration and when checking the cabin, cabin crew are trained to switch their focus from 'warm and friendly' customer service to safety and security in order to make sure that everyone is securely seated and has the information they need. If you are sitting by an exit, you'll probably get an extra briefing from one of the crew to make sure that you are able to open the door in the very unlikely event that you need to. Again, it's not because they expect you to have to do it, but because it's safer to make sure that you can. If you're not happy, ask questions or ask to move seats – they'll be able to arrange that for you.

During the safety demonstration, pay attention and make sure you know where your life jacket is, what the brace position is, where your nearest exit is, how to get there and how to open it. Then concentrate on something else; you've done everything you can to make yourself as safe as possible. You are now in the safest category of airline passenger – the ones who are prepared!

## How well trained are pilots?

People tend to ask this question because they are anxious about not being in control and having to trust complete strangers to fly an aircraft. This is a completely understandable way to think, but as you read the other chapters in this book, you will realize that there are techniques you can use to control anxious thoughts like this one.

The minimum qualification that a pilot must hold in order to fly aircraft with paying passengers or cargo is a Commercial Pilot's Licence (CPL). To obtain a CPL, a pilot must either gain sufficient experience in light aircraft, or flying military aircraft, or take a full-time course of flying and ground training. In all cases, pilots have to pass a large number of written examinations on subjects such as aviation law, meteorology and navigation. They also have to pass two flight tests, one flying in visual conditions and one to demonstrate that they can safely fly using the aircraft instruments in all weather conditions.

Once pilots have a CPL, they apply to airlines who use very rigorous selection procedures to identify the best candidates. Before they can fly a passenger aircraft, pilots must do a technical course and pass a written examination on the aircraft they will be flying. They also have to complete a training course in the simulator covering normal flying and emergency procedures. They must pass a practical test in the simulator before they can fly the actual aircraft. They then spend a period of time flying with a training captain until they pass a final test and can fly as a first officer.

Pilots are probably the most supervised and tested professionals on earth. Every year they must pass two tests in the simulator, two written examinations and complete a supervised normal flight. They are also under constant observation by the pilots they fly with. Each flight is conducted by two pilots, a captain and a first officer, and both must prove at every test that they can fly the aircraft without the other. In day-to-day flying, they take it in turns to fly, so the captain may fly from London to Paris and the first officer will fly back to London. The captain is the senior and usually more experienced pilot and is ultimately responsible for conducting the flight safely.

After gaining a minimum amount of experience, a pilot with a CPL takes another practical test and upgrades his or her licence to an Airline Transport Pilot's Licence (ATPL). Eventually, once he or she has an ATPL and sufficient experience, a first officer will be promoted to the position of captain.

### Are take-offs and landings more dangerous than the rest of the flight?

Very often people tell us that the take-off or landing is the part of a flight which they worry about most. This might be because they are the noisiest parts of the flight, the stages where you feel most acceleration, pressing you into your seat or where you begin to feel as if you are descending or – for take-off – simply because it's the point at which you really start to fly.

A large part of pilot training concentrates on take-offs and landings and on what to do if anything unexpected happens. It is also a requirement that pilots have to carry out a minimum number of landings in a set period of time. In the UK this is three landings in 90 days. If they have not done this, then they have to go and practise in the simulator before they are allowed to fly again.

Remember that incredibly few accidents happen when flying. Within this very small number, it is possible that a greater proportion happen during take-off or landing. This is probably because these are the parts of flight when the aircraft is closest to the ground and to other aircraft. It is similar to the way in which most road accidents take place at junctions, where cars are closer to each other and to road boundaries.

If you are particularly anxious about take-off or landing, try and use these times to practise your relaxation techniques.

## How does an aeroplane fly?

We find that people most often ask this question because they worry either that something so large shouldn't be able to 'defy gravity' and fly, or that if the engines do develop a fault the aircraft will 'fall'. If you are one of these people, use the information here to develop an understanding of how aircraft fly so that you can construct a new way of thinking, as described in Chapter 7. This is the way in which all aircraft fly, from the largest A380 'double decker' to the smallest two-seat trainer.

An aeroplane flies because of the way in which four forces act together. These are weight, lift, thrust and drag. When an aeroplane is flying in a straight line and maintaining the same height and speed, the four forces balance each other. (For those of you who use or remember some physics, this is Newton's First Law of Motion.) This is shown in Figure 9.1.

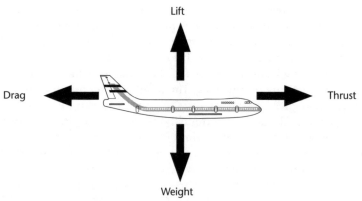

**Figure 9.1 The four forces**

We will briefly describe how each of these forces works in a way that does not assume that you currently know or use any physics or aero-dynamics. The books listed under 'Other sources of help' at the end of this book contain more scientific explanations if you need them.

*Weight* is the effect of the earth's gravity and if it was the only force acting would pull the aircraft towards the ground. The size of this 'pull' depends simply on how much mass (material) the aircraft has.

*Lift* is a force generated by air flowing over the wings and acts mainly in the opposite direction to weight. If the aircraft is flying in a straight line and the amount of lift is the same as the amount of weight, then the aircraft stays at the same height. This is important to know: it's not the engines that stop an aircraft being pulled to the ground, it's the lift generated by the wings. Without engines, an aircraft becomes a glider and will descend slowly, covering about a mile over ground every time it descends 500 feet. Figure 9.2 shows a cross-section of a typical aircraft wing, indicating the airflow over and below it.

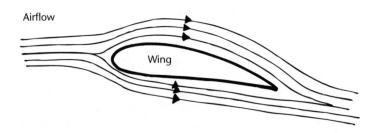

Airflow

Wing

**Figure 9.2  Airflow around an aircraft wing**

The science behind the way in which a wing generates lift depends on Bernoulli's Theorem, which is explained in some of the books in the reading list. The wing is shaped so that air flowing over the top of it has to travel faster than air flowing below it, because it has to go further to get from the front to the back of the wing. Air which travels faster exerts less pressure on the wing. The result is lower pressure above the wing and higher pressure below the wing. The wing is 'pushed' up from below and 'sucked' up from above. You can see this for yourself by holding a piece of paper in front of your mouth. If you blow across the top surface, it should rise because air is travelling faster over the top surface, creating lower pressure which 'sucks' the paper up.

The amount of lift which a wing creates will increase if:

- air flows faster over the wing (the aircraft increases speed);

- the wing is more curved;
- the wing is thicker.

Large aircraft normally fly at high speeds so that air flows over the wing very quickly, creating large amounts of lift. When an aircraft needs to fly more slowly, flaps and slats are used to make the wing more curved, again creating more lift.

*Thrust* is produced by the engines and pulls the aircraft forward, either along the ground or through the air. Air enters at the front of an engine and is compressed. Some of it is passed to a central core, where it is combined with fuel and burns at very high temperatures. This hot air and the unburnt cold air are pushed very quickly out of the back of the engine. This in turn pushes the engines, and therefore the aircraft, forward (Newton's Third Law of Motion, if you want to look at the science). If you blow up a party balloon and let go before tying the neck, the same thing happens.

*Drag* is generated by the friction that happens when anything moves through air. You can feel this if you stick your hand (carefully!) out of a moving car window: if you turn your palm towards the air, your hand will be pushed back quite forcefully. If you now turn it so that your hand is flat, there's less resistance. Drag tends to act in the opposite direction to thrust, so aircraft are designed with 'streamlined' shapes to keep this to an absolute minimum. As drag increases, the engines need to produce more thrust to counter it.

## What's that noise?

People who are anxious pay a great deal of attention to the sights and sounds around them, reading 'danger' into them or looking for signs that there may be a problem. This is a completely understandable reaction, but unfortunately it is not helpful: being extra attentive actually adds to your physical tension, makes you think negatively and increases your anxiety. You will often be more relaxed if you follow the advice in Chapter 7 and distract yourself or practise a relaxation technique. However, if you do begin to worry about a particular noise, one way to tackle that thought is to know what the noise or sound really is. You will hear a wide range of noises in an aircraft that you probably will not hear anywhere else. We will try and explain the more common ones here.

### Engine noises

The thrust required from the engines varies continuously through a flight. When taking off and during the first part of the climb, the engines will be producing a lot of thrust and will be quite loud. Normally, at about 1,500 feet, the pilots will reduce the thrust required and this can cause the engine noise to change quite suddenly. Particularly in Europe and the USA, it is unusual to be able to climb all the way to cruising altitude in one step; there may be a number of quite sudden changes in engine noise as the aircraft climbs and then stays level for a while before climbing again. The sudden changes in engine noise often cause people to think that the engines have developed a fault, so it may be sensible to remind yourself just before take-off that the engines will be very noisy to start with but will probably become quieter quite suddenly, shortly after you leave the ground.

There will probably be several sudden changes in engine noise while the aircraft is climbing. At the same time you may feel acceleration pushes you into your seat as engine noise increases, or even a slight floating sensation when thrust reduces suddenly and the engines become quiet. This can cause a false sensation of falling backwards, which worries many people. If it is a day when you can see outside, you will see that the aircraft is climbing or flying level. If you are flying through cloud, remind yourself that rapid changes in engine thrust often confuse your body and send false signals to the brain. Climbing this way may seem uncomfortable, but remember that it actually helps to maintain the very large distances between aircraft around busy airports and therefore makes you even safer. The same thing applies when you are descending towards your arrival airport. Even when the aircraft is cruising, the engine noise may change from time to time as the pilots need to fly at a faster or slower speed, or turn anti-icing systems on or off.

Descending requires much less thrust and is often carried out with the engines at 'idle' (just like a car engine waiting at a junction). This means a lot less noise and again can happen quite suddenly. Like the climb, the descent usually happens in steps and engine noises will change each time the aircraft levels off. Particularly in the last stages of a flight, aircraft need to be flown at accurate speeds to fit in with other aircraft near the airport. This can result in frequent changes in engine noise. After landing, the pilots may use reverse thrust to help slow the aircraft and this is very noisy. What happens is that the engine covers open to form a cone which directs most of the air which would normally exit at the back of the engine forward. This works to push back on the aircraft and slow it down, but reduces the noise shielding around the engine, hence the loud noise.

If there is a loud 'bang' from an engine, it may mean that that engine has been damaged. This is incredibly rare. Aircraft are only allowed to carry passengers if they are built so that any damage to an engine is contained within that engine and they can safely fly with one engine not operating (aircraft with four engines have to be able to fly with only two operating). Engines are self-contained and any damage will be controlled without damaging surrounding areas. If it does happen, the pilots will control the aircraft and keep it flying safely. They will then plan where to go – normally the nearest suitable airport – and brief the cabin crew about the new plan. They will then talk to the passengers and explain what's happening, but it might take 15 minutes or even a little longer before this happens. You might be delayed but you will be safe.

### External noises

Lots of other noises are caused by changes in the airflow outside the aircraft. There's more of this type of noise as the aircraft speed increases and less as it slows down. Other external noises include the sound of the landing gear going up into the fuselage after take-off or down for landing, the operation of hydraulic pumps to move control surfaces or the movement of speedbrakes, slats or flaps. Incidentally, on some aircraft, one of the hydraulic pumps sometimes used on the ground sounds like a dog barking!

### Internal noises

There are a wide range of cabin noises too. Cabin panels and lockers have to be made of strong fireproof materials with a degree of flexibility, but this means they creak! Galleys are full of trolleys, catering boxes and trays which rattle. Different air-conditioning systems make different noises in the cabin too.

## What about turbulence?

Turbulence is one of the topics that comes up most frequently when we talk to people who are afraid of flying. That is understandable because flying through turbulence is uncomfortable for everyone on board. The effect can be to send a false signal to the brain that we are in trouble, which will raise anxiety levels and make us hypervigilant, seeing 'danger' in every aircraft movement or cabin crew action. It can cause fear because it seems unexplained and unpredictable; it may feel as though the aeroplane is out of control. Turbulence can also be disorientating and make you feel ill. Newspaper headlines that talk about 'air pockets' and 'aircraft falling' do not help either. It is worth mentioning here that because turbulence is uncomfortable and worrying, its occurrence has a tendency to become a vivid memory. You are much more likely to remember the part of the flight when you flew through turbulence than the rest of it, even though it might be less than 30 minutes of an eight-hour flight. This means that you become more likely to anticipate flying through turbulence on your next flight, which will make you even more anxious.

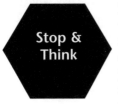

**Stop &
Think**

Before you read the rest of the information on turbulence, make a few notes on exactly what makes you anxious about it. Is it your fear of damage to the aircraft, worrying that you will panic or something else? Once you've read the information that follows, see if you can create new ways of thinking about it. There is more on how to do this in Chapter 7.

### What causes turbulence?

Aircraft fly through air and they will be affected if the air is changing direction rapidly or suddenly starts to move faster or to slow down. Because air is a mixture of gases, you can't normally see it. If you're on a boat, you can see where the waves are larger or more frequent and know which areas will be most likely to create a bumpy ride. This is very similar to the effect that air has on an aircraft. Turbulence in air is caused either by the weather or by other aircraft.

### Weather that causes turbulence

Clouds associated with showers and storms – cumulus and cumulo-nimbus clouds – sit at the top of very large columns of air which is rising very quickly. Inside the cloud, water condenses into large rain droplets and starts to fall, causing the air to move in many directions. Outside the column of rising air, air moves rapidly down to replace the air which has risen towards the cloud. This means that in and around thunderstorms, very heavy showers and large cumulus clouds, air is rapidly changing direction and there is likely to be turbulence.

Turbulence can also happen where there are no clouds. At many places in the atmosphere there are long horizontal tubes of fast-moving air known as 'jet streams'. These can actually be very useful, as the air inside them is usually smooth or only slightly turbulent; if you fly back from America to Europe, a helpful jet stream can reduce the duration of your flight by an hour or more. However, the air around jet streams is not very smooth and flying near small jet streams or getting into or out of the large ones which help long flights, will mean flying through some turbulence.

## *Avoiding turbulence*

When planning a flight, pilots will check weather forecasts to look for stormy areas and will either take extra fuel to fly around them, plan to fly at a higher level to avoid them or arrange to fly a different route to their destination. Aviation weather forecasts are more specific than those on radio and television but no forecast is perfect, so all flights carry extra or 'contingency' fuel so that the pilots can avoid any unexpected areas of bad weather. Modern aircraft are equipped with radar systems that will detect areas of storms and turbulence and pilots will avoid flying through these.

When pilots do fly into unexpected turbulence, they tell air traffic control and other aircraft so that everyone else knows where the area of turbulence is. Often, they'll then climb or descend and this will usually mean getting back to smooth flight. If you are on a flight that becomes bumpy, it probably won't be for more than 30 to 40 minutes. The most common exception to this is flights from North America to Europe, particularly at night, where the route will normally plan to use the helpful jet streams to make the flight as short as possible. Flying in these jet streams may mean that the flight is slightly turbulent for most of the time crossing the Atlantic. If it's going to be very turbulent, pilots plan another route.

Some turbulence is caused by other aircraft, in a very similar way to the wake caused by a boat on water. This is one of the reasons why aircraft are always flown with a minimum distance between each one.

## *Will turbulence damage the aircraft?*

This is one of the things about turbulence that we find worries people most. Before they are certified to carry passengers, aircraft manufacturers must demonstrate that their aircraft is stronger than required to cope with extreme turbulence. Most aircraft will never encounter anything more than mild or moderate turbulence. Remember that most turbulence is predictable, so most flights will not encounter much turbulence at all. Any turbulence you do fly through will not damage the aircraft. Overall, *turbulence is uncomfortable, but not dangerous*. It may be so uncomfortable that it can mean your body sends a false signal to your brain saying that you are in trouble. This is yet another way in which anxiety may increase during turbulence. In Chapter 10 you will find a comprehensive list reminding you of the techniques that will be most helpful if turbulence increases your anxiety.

## So why do the wings bend and flex in turbulence?

If you look out at the wings of an aircraft, particularly on a bumpy flight, you will often see the wing tips moving up and down. Pilots and engineers call this 'flexing'. We often find that this makes people think that the wings will snap or break. This is a completely rational way to think, but aircraft wings are designed to be flexible. This actually makes them stronger than if they were built to be absolutely rigid. Flexible structures are often stronger than rigid ones. Tall buildings and bridges are also designed to be flexible and will sway in strong winds; they are stronger that way.

## What do the crew do when it's turbulent?

We often hear that watching how the cabin crew react to turbulence can make people more anxious. This is a very understandable way to think about what you might see, because the crew will change from emphasizing their role in serving customers to considering safety first. This is not because turbulence is dangerous to the aircraft, but because passengers could possibly fall and loose objects or hot liquids might move or spill. Their behaviour has to change, in the same way that a policeman would behave very differently when giving you directions or moving you away from an incident in a public place. You may notice that cabin crew start to use more assertive body language and speech and even move more quickly. Quite often any trolleys will be pushed back into the galleys and stowed. The crew's aim is to make sure that everyone is safely seated with their seat belt fastened and that anything loose is put away so that it can't cause any problems.

Think of the way in which the crew's behaviour changes as a way of making sure that you are as comfortable as possible.

One of the other comments we hear is that it often takes a long time for pilots to explain what's happening if the aircraft flies into turbulence. That's not because they don't care or because they are busy trying to 'save' the aeroplane. Different airlines have varied procedures; they might advise pilots not to make announcements in certain situations but to leave it to the cabin crew. The pilots may also be busy talking to air traffic control and other aircraft to see if there is a smoother route or height to fly at.

## Why's the aircraft shuddering?

People often say that they become anxious when they feel the aircraft begin to shudder. The most common reason for this to happen is that the pilots are using the speedbrakes to slow the aeroplane down or to descend more rapidly. Just after take-off you may feel some aircraft shudder as the landing gear is retracted. This is because the wheels are still rotating very quickly and they rub against strips in the wheel bays designed to stop this. This rubbing can make the aircraft shudder for up to two or three minutes.

## What do they mean by 'technical problem'?

We've often heard people mention that they've been delayed because of a 'technical problem' and that this has understandably made them anxious about getting on an aeroplane that may have a fault. People have also told us that it seems to happen more frequently to aeroplanes than when they're driving a car.

If you are told that there has been a technical problem with your flight, it could be anything from needing a light bulb or wheel changed to a major fault that needs a team of engineers to fix. How much information you get will depend on where you are and what the airline's policy is. Some tend not to tell you what the fault is because they don't want to make people anxious, others often give you more technical information than you need or even want.

The first thing to think about if this happens is that this is a fault which has been found before you get on the aircraft, and that the engineers and pilots will not allow the flight to happen until they are convinced it is safe. Each aircraft has a list of faults with which it can fly safely; if the engineers have checked that the problem is one of these faults and that there are no others, then the flight will be safe. This is a bit like accepting that you can safely drive your car if the radio is broken, but not if the brakes don't work.

A typical technical problem that might delay a modern passenger aeroplane would be a fault in one of the three navigation systems. If this happens, the engineers or pilots must check that both other systems work correctly before each flight. One system on its own would navigate safely, but passenger aircraft always start a flight with at least one back-up system. If a fault occurs that isn't on the approved list, it must be fixed before the aeroplane is allowed to fly. This can delay your flight, particularly if the engineers need to carry out detailed checks to make sure that the fault has been fixed correctly. Alternatively, it might mean that your flight is delayed until another aircraft becomes available.

Remember that finding the fault before flying is a good thing, and that the aeroplane won't be allowed to fly until it's been either fixed or checked against the approved list of 'safe' faults. You might be delayed but you will be safe.

Faults seem to happen more often to aircraft than cars because aircraft get checked more frequently and they have more back-up systems. If you have a car, how often do you check the oil level and tyre pressures or look all round it for damage? Either a pilot or an engineer walks round an aircraft to check for damage and checks the oil levels before every flight, and engineers check tyre pressures at least every two days. This means that faults are identified as soon as they happen and are checked before the next flight. Most aircraft have more than one system for braking, navigating and providing electrical power. That means that there are more systems which can develop faults. However, only one of each needs to work for the aircraft to fly safely.

## What are those engineers doing?

If you see one or more engineers around the aircraft you're about to board, it's most likely that they're carrying out the pre-flight inspection. This has to be done before each flight to make sure that there are no new faults or damage. On some aircraft, this can mean opening the engine covers or 'cowls' to check oil levels. The engineers may also be performing tasks such as changing wheels or external lights.

## That aircraft looks dirty or scratched. Is it safe?

Many people tell us that they worry about getting on an aircraft that looks dirty or scratched because they think it might mean that the aircraft is old or unsafe. As we have suggested, you can use the techniques in Chapter 7 and the information given in this chapter to develop a more realistic way of thinking about this.

Every part of every aircraft is licensed only for a specified number of flights or flying hours. These limits are set after very rigorous tests which establish how long each part can be safely used. Any part must be replaced well before it is likely to develop a fault. The whole aircraft will be inspected at frequent intervals to check for 'wear and tear', which must then be repaired. However old an aircraft is – and they can safely fly for decades – it will only carry passengers if engineers are satisfied that it is still safe to do so.

If you watch an aircraft at the departure gate, you'll see it is surrounded by trucks loading baggage, catering or fuel and often has moveable steps to allow the crew and engineers access. This is the main reason why, if you look closely, most aircraft will have a few bumps and scratches. Just like a car, paint scratches and small dents aren't dangerous, but an engineer must check each one to make sure that there is no other damage. Each aircraft has a record of dents which have been checked and measured, and part of the inspection carried out before each flight checks for any new ones. These must be examined and recorded before the next flight.

Particularly if the aircraft has recently landed on a wet runway, it may be dirty, just like your car. It may not look very pretty, especially if most of the aircraft is white (if you have a white car, how dirty does it look after driving along a wet motorway?), but it is safe. If there is too much dirt, the pilot or engineer who carries out the pre-flight inspection will make sure the aircraft is cleaned.

## What happens if ...?

We find that when people ask questions about what can go wrong with a flight, they are already using their very active imagination to picture an accident or frightening event. Having an active imagination is great – if it is working for your benefit. If it is helping you to imagine traumatic events, then try using the information here to imagine a safe outcome. For example, you may think that if an engine fails, the aeroplane will crash. If so, remember that aircraft have to be able to fly safely in the event of this happening, while every six months pilots practise what to do in such an event. Use the complete answer below to find out what is likely to happen if an engine does fail, taking time to sit down and imagine a safe landing after an engine failure. Do this for any of the 'what if ...' questions in this section that you worry about.

### What if an engine fails?

This is one of the 'what if ...' questions we are asked most frequently. To start with, try and remember that it is very unlikely ever to happen to you. Modern passenger aircraft have to demonstrate a very low level of engine failures before they're allowed to fly. Having said that, engine failures do happen. They hardly ever lead to people getting hurt.

If an engine does stop working properly, the pilot who is flying will have made sure that the aeroplane is flying in the correct direction and climbing safely. If necessary, both pilots will check with each other to confirm which engine has failed and what the problem was. Sometimes, it is possible at this stage to restart the failed engine. Even if this does happen, the pilots will normally land as soon as possible to get the fault checked and fixed, rather than continue with a long flight. If the engine cannot be restarted, one pilot will follow a checklist to make sure that the failed engine is no longer supplied with fuel and limit any further damage. The same pilot will also start any back-up systems, such as additional electrical supply and air-conditioning systems, in order to make sure these are available if necessary. The pilot flying the aeroplane will normally be using the autopilot to fly at this stage (the autopilot is a set of computers that will automatically fly an aircraft at the height and speed and in the direction selected by the pilots. It is used so that pilots can monitor exactly what the aircraft is doing without having to concentrate on physically flying it all the time. It makes flying safer and more accurate), and will tell air traffic control what the problem is and start flying towards a suitable airfield. Once the aircraft is safe and flying towards an airfield, the pilots will brief the cabin crew.

All of this takes up to 15 minutes to deal with safely, so it may be a while before one of the pilots makes an announcement to explain what has happened. You may notice unusual noises, or find that the cabin crew suddenly stop the in-flight service, well before the pilots tell you what has happened. Cabin crew are trained not to interrupt the pilots, so they may not know any more than you to start with.

Landing with an engine shut down is another skill that pilots practise every six months, and it is also something that the autopilot can do at most large airports. To a pilot, it is not very different from a normal landing once the failed engine has been properly secured. Because it happens so rarely in real life, an aircraft landing after an engine failure will usually get an escort of fire engines once it has landed and as it taxis to the parking position.

If the pilots decide to land somewhere other than the planned destination, they will usually be able to alert airline ground staff by radio on the way. Over most of Europe, it doesn't take more than 30 or 40 minutes to fly to and land at a suitable airport, so the airline may not have had much chance to set up arrangements for passengers. If it is safe, you may even find that you have to stay on the aircraft for a while after it parks. This would be a good time to practise your distraction and relaxation techniques if you can. If it's appropriate, you could talk to the people around you, who will have been just as anxious as you.

Overall, such an event is very unlikely to happen to you. If it does happen, you will be safe. You may have to wait to find out what's happened, you will be delayed and probably initially end up somewhere you didn't plan to be. Eventually the airline will get you safely to your destination or return home.

## What if the pilots become ill?

You may be asking this question because you're worried about who is going to land the aircraft if one of the pilots can't. All passenger aircraft with more than 12 seats have to be flown by two or more pilots, one of whom can land the aircraft on his or her own. In the very unlikely event that both pilots become ill, modern passenger aircraft have automatic pilots which can actually land at major airports and stop on the runway without any pilot action. Senior cabin crew are trained in how to use the radio to ask for help and will be able to use the autopilot to land the aircraft following instructions over the radio. There is often a qualified pilot among the passengers anyway.

So that you know how unlikely it is that a pilot will fall ill, here is some information on how pilots are medically checked. In the UK, pilots undergo a medical check every year. This is designed to pick up any health problems well before they might lead to incapacitating sickness in flight. If any problems are detected, they must be treated before a pilot can fly again. If they can't be treated, the pilot is no longer able to fly. You might like to know that there are people who run marathons who cannot meet the medical standards required to be a commercial pilot.

## What happens if there is smoke in the cabin?

The thought of seeing smoke on board an aircraft is a frightening one. As with most of these 'what if ...' situations, we'd like you to start by remembering that it's unlikely to happen to you. When it has happened in modern passenger aircraft, most have landed safely and most passengers and crew have evacuated safely.

Cabin crew and pilots are regularly trained in dealing with the most likely causes of smoke in aircraft. These include passengers smoking in toilets, smoking ovens in the galley, heat in toilet waste bins and smoke in overhead lockers. Aircraft carry very effective fire-fighting equipment and have multiple automatic detection systems.

If smoke is detected, the crew may need to move you out of the way quickly to get to the source and put it out. One of the cabin crew will tell the pilots what is happening and they may decide to land as soon as possible. If there's a lot of smoke in the cabin, you may find that the passenger oxygen masks are released from the cabin ceiling so that you can breathe safely.

This is another time when you may see the crew's behaviour change from warm and friendly to focused on what they have to do. They are well trained in dealing with smoke and will be able to deal with it quickly and effectively, but they may not have time to reassure you while they do so.

## I worry when I see television reports or newspaper articles about flying incidents

We have often talked to people who are made very anxious by reports such as 'Aircraft plummets 20,000 feet' or 'Plane aborts take-off'. These headlines, and the reports and television pictures that often go with them, fuel fear and anxiety for obvious reasons.

The first step in dealing with anxieties about reports like these is to make sure that you keep a sense of proportion. Did you ever see a headline saying '40,000 flights arrived safely at Heathrow last month'? Remember that the media do not report the thousands of flights which safely take place every day.

There are some very rare occasions when the media reports accidents which have resulted in people being hurt. If you look at such reports carefully, though, they are often a dramatic description of the way in which the back-up systems in an aircraft have worked safely. For example, the headline 'Aircraft plummets 20,000 feet' would probably relate to an incident where the main cabin pressurization system and its back-up both developed faults. In this case, the next back-up system, individual oxygen masks, functioned correctly and everyone continued to breathe. The pilots will have descended quickly and safely to a height where additional oxygen was no longer needed and the masks could be removed. It was probably a frightening experience but the aircraft was safe at all times. Remember that headlines such as 'Aircraft oxygen masks worked and plane landed safely' do not sell newspapers or encourage people to watch television!

## But what if the worst happens?

Even if you're imagining a 'what if ...' situation that we haven't covered, the airlines, aircraft manufacturers and regulating authorities will have thought of it and provided training for pilots and cabin crew. The most common comment from crews involved in this type of situation is 'That was just the way we practised in training'.

We sometimes find that people who seek treatment for fear of flying will ask questions such as 'What would it be like to die in an incident on an aircraft?' In our experience, people who express such anxieties are probably primarily afraid of death and dying, though it presents as a fear of flying. They may have a vivid mental picture of being involved in one of the very rare accidents they may have heard about and become fixated on catastrophe. If you find yourself persistently thinking and worrying about this, working with a psychologist is likely to be the most effective way to manage these difficult and intrusive thoughts.

## And finally ...

This chapter contains a lot of information and we hope you've found it useful. Remember that if you don't find the answer to your specific question in this chapter, you should be able to challenge any anxious thoughts using the general information at the start. Use the information in this chapter which is relevant to you, combined with the techniques explained in Chapter 7, to create new ways of thinking about flying.

# 10

# Helpful hints and tips

This chapter summarizes the most important things you may need to remind yourself of before and during a flight. Some are hints and tips to help you plan your trip, while others are prompts to help you make the best use of your new psychological skills. We have included a section which considers what you might do if you plan to fly and decide not to, whether before travelling to the airport, at the airport or boarding the aircraft. This may seem rather pessimistic, but remember that we do not expect you to fail! People often tell us that they worry about what to do if they decide not to travel at the last minute, and some people even find it easier to get on the aeroplane if they know there is a constructive plan should they become too anxious and decide not to fly. The section is here to help you find additional sources of help if at any stage you decide you do not yet have all the skills you need to be able to fly with reduced anxiety. If you would like to think about planning what to do if you decide you need more skills in order to fly confidently, read through it. If not, skip it and just look at the lists of hints and tips.

The first four lists may seem quite obvious and not related to the techniques in this book. They summarize the administration and planning required to make your flight go smoothly. We often find that people are easily distracted when they are preparing for any activity that makes them anxious. This increases your level of anxiety when you are preparing to travel and may mean that you are likely to forget something important, which will make your journey more stressful than it needs to be. We have started with planning and preparation so that you have an outline to work from to prepare for your journey. The later lists include one to use if you are travelling with a sympathetic companion, and others which remind you of the techniques and skills you now have to overcome your fear of flying.

## A final case study

Now that you have had a chance to discover the skills, information and techniques in the main part of this book, we have included one final case study to show you how one person came to understand his own fear of flying and select and practise the skills that eventually helped him to overcome his fear. As with all the other case studies in this book, we have changed any personal details.

Joshua remembered many happy holiday flights with his parents as a child and had flown confidently as an adult until he reached his mid-thirties. He then started to become increasingly anxious about flying. Eventually he refused to plan a holiday to America with his wife and two children because he was too anxious to fly. He could not explain his fear to his family and they repeatedly tried to persuade him to change his decision.

During one conversation with his wife, Joshua started to explain that he didn't understand how anyone could control an aircraft and said that he didn't want to 'strap myself into an aluminium tube which I have no idea how to control'. She suggested that he learn to fly at their local airport. He took his first flying lesson and his instructor let him handle the controls to make the small aeroplane climb, turn and descend. Flushed with success, Joshua returned home and booked the holiday to America, much to his family's surprise and delight!

There was time for one more flying lesson before they went to America but unfortunately, when Joshua arrived, the aircraft he was supposed to fly had developed a technical fault. He spent the time in the flying club lounge listening to stories of 'near misses' from other students and pilots. Two days later, the family flew to America.

Joshua spent the flight thinking about the tales he had heard two days previously and began to imagine many things that could go wrong during the eight-hour flight to their destination. He started to watch the crew for any signs of anxiety and when he saw one female crew member look worried, followed her into the galley to find out what was wrong. He didn't really believe her explanation that she had lost her mobile phone, and spent the rest of the flight closely watching the crew and listening for any 'unusual' noises. He even quizzed one of the cabin crew on the qualifications held by the pilots. His wife tried everything she could think of to persuade him to relax, but he remained anxious for the whole flight.

The holiday was spoilt by Joshua's constant worry about the flight home. He decided to 'manage' his fear by having several alcoholic drinks. After a very unpleasant start to the flight, he fell into a restless doze. When they returned home, Joshua vowed never to fly again, feeling deeply ashamed. When the time came to plan the next family holiday, Joshua stammered through an attempt to explain why he did not want to fly. His wife insisted that he should get himself 'sorted out'. He consulted his GP, who referred him to a psychologist.

Working with the psychologist, Joshua started to explore why he had become anxious about flying after many years of confidently travelling by air. He was surprised, and reassured, to learn that this is actually a pattern which many people who become fearful of flying experience. He started to think of it as something that had developed as he became more aware of possible problems and matured from the 'over-confident teenager' he had once been. Joshua found this especially comforting as it reduced the shame and embarrassment he felt at being anxious about flying.

During his therapy, Joshua began to realize that one factor which added to his anxious thoughts about flying was the hours he had spent in his early thirties watching television documentaries about aircraft incidents. This had been at about the same time as news reports of an aircraft accident he could still describe in detail. The psychologist suggested that Joshua had learnt to associate flying with the frightening incidents covered in the documentaries and news reports. When they worked on identifying Joshua's negative thoughts, they discovered that he thought of large passenger aircraft as 'dangerous' and 'likely to crash'. Joshua had probably been able to enjoy his flying lesson because it was in such a different aeroplane from those involved in the television programmes he had seen. Together they worked on challenging these thoughts in the way we describe in Chapter 7. In between sessions, Joshua practised realistic thinking and relaxation exercises.

In later sessions of therapy, Joshua and the psychologist also worked on other thoughts associated with the way in which he considered the flying involved 'handing over control' to pilots he did not know and could not trust. They used information similar to that given in Chapter 9 to challenge these thoughts. Gradually the psychologist started to encourage Joshua to complete 'homework' similar to the graded practice we describe in Chapter 7. He started with a return visit to his local airfield and later took his wife to lunch at the airport they had used to fly to America. Eventually, Joshua and his wife flew to Paris for a short break after a session where they had both worked with the psychologist to decide how she could be most helpful when they flew together. Both flights went well, although Joshua was slightly tense; his wife helped to remind him to practise the relaxation skills he had learnt. Two weeks later, Joshua flew alone to Edinburgh to visit some friends.

Flying will never be Joshua's favourite form of travel. With the help of the techniques he learnt through working with a psychologist, he describes his anxiety as 'manageable' and can fly reasonably comfortably as required. The family go on holiday once a year and Joshua is able to enjoy being away without worrying about the flight home.

## If you decide not to fly yet

If you have decided not to travel this time, whether you have been unable to book a ticket, got as far as the airport, or even been approaching the aircraft before turning back, you may find that you become quite critical of yourself for not travelling. If you have worked through this book, it is likely that you have made some progress, so start by giving yourself credit for what you have achieved. Reading parts of this book means that you have shown courage and motivation to take steps to overcome your fear of flying. If you have booked a ticket or driven to the airport when you might not have done so before, then you have indeed made progress. You have more information about fear of flying, which is a good start to overcoming it. Remember the way in which we described how to challenge negative thoughts about flying earlier in this book? Use those techniques to make realistic challenges to any critical thoughts you may be having if you decided not to travel.

## Things to consider when you plan a flight

Think about these as you start to plan and book your flight in order to make sure it is less stressful for you and goes as smoothly as possible.

### Planning

- Why are you going? Think of the main incentives for you and what you stand to gain and enjoy. Think about the holiday, what you will achieve on the business trip or who you are going to meet. Concentrate on the things that will motivate you to take the flight and make a note of them.
- Avoid delaying or putting off making your booking. The sooner you do it, the quicker you can focus on your goals and the skills you will need to achieve them. The worst thing that can happen is that you do not fly.
- What techniques in this book do you think will work best? List them for yourself and make a note of them. Plan some time to practise them before you go and think about when you're going to use them on your flight.
- Plan ahead: how are you going to get to the airport? Will you be on

your own or travelling with someone? Be there on time or ahead of time. Get organized so that you feel more in control. Avoid leaving things until the last moment, when you may increase your stress levels – this will not help you on your flight.

- Do you need any vaccinations? Remember to organize these well ahead of travel.
- If you haven't used a particular airport before, look at its website if you can. Plan where to get dropped off or park, and where to check in or drop off your luggage. Make sure you plan to eat before leaving for the airport. It may be a while before you eat on the flight and you may find that you do not want to eat when travelling. Find out where to check in and what you can take through security in cabin baggage. If you can check in online before you go to the airport, that often means less time and hassle at the airport itself. Many airlines provide automatic check-in machines at airports and have details of how to use these on their websites. Airport websites will have details of what facilities will be available in the departure area.
- How are you going to get from your arrival airport to your final destination? Again, plan ahead.
- Who else is going? Do they know that you have a fear of flying? Can they help you use the skills and techniques you want to try? Should you share the ideas that you have learnt about your fear and how to manage it with them?
- What can you do to make the experience less stressful? Even if you're travelling in economy class, most airports have executive lounges which, for a fee, offer a quiet and more relaxed place to be before flying. If there is a meal on the flight, do you need to request a special option to suit your dietary requirements, such as being vegetarian? Do you need to take your own food?
- What do you need to do before you go? Try and make sure you will not have to rush around too much before travelling. This will make you more susceptible to anxiety and even to a panic attack. Put time aside to deal with the essentials and accept that anything else will have to wait until you get back.
- Can you plan something enjoyable for when you return to help your motivation to succeed? If it is a challenging business trip, try to plan something while you are away as well, even if it's only some time spent not working.

## What to pack?

There are numerous travel books which will tell you what you need to take. The following lists are designed to remind you to think about the things that will help you reduce your anxiety. The first considers what you might want to include in your carry-on cabin baggage, the second considers hold baggage or large suitcases. Make sure that you check with the airport or airline that your cabin bag is of an acceptable size.

If you are flying from the UK, and in some other parts of the world, you can only carry a limited amount of liquids, toiletries and so on in your cabin baggage in a sealed plastic bag. Anything over this allowance will have to go in your hold baggage. Check with the airport website before you go what the rules are, and see the separate checklist on liquids for ideas on what might be useful. You will always be able to take any medication that you need into the cabin and it is useful to take a copy of your prescription with you. The sealed plastic bag should fit inside your cabin bag.

### Carry-on luggage

- A copy of this book!
- Any medication you need for the journey. Remember travel sickness remedies if you need them.
- The obvious things which we are all prone to forget: travel documents (passport, tickets or e-tickets), itinerary, spectacles/sunglasses, wallet, mobile phone, cash in local and foreign currencies, important contact numbers, a pen and notebook. Remember to organize travel visas, if necessary, well beforehand. If you have an e-ticket, make sure that you have whatever identification or payment card you need to retrieve it at check-in.
- Snack food – low blood sugar levels will only make anxiety worse, so have with you some sensible snack food that is easy to eat – cereal bars, nuts, dried fruit.
- Anything you have decided to use as distractions for the flight – crosswords, puzzles, Sudoku, books, newspapers, music, DVD player. But avoid planning to do anything too taxing or stressful. Take work with you if you have room – it might be a good distraction – but do not put yourself under pressure to get it done. You may find that it's not the right thing to concentrate on. Remember that you will not be able to use electronic equipment when the seat-belt signs are switched on.
- As long as it fits in, take anything important in your cabin bag. That way you know you will have it when you arrive, even if it takes a

while for your hold baggage to emerge. Some flyers take a change of underclothes and other essentials in case their main luggage goes missing!

## Checked-in (hold) luggage

- A back-up copy of this book, if you are prone to losing things.
- Distractions for the return flight – music, DVDs, puzzles, etc.
- Clothes, gifts, non-essential work items and toiletries.
- Something to remind you why you're taking this trip and how you are going to reward yourself when you get back – even if it is only a note in your suitcase.
- A spare plastic bag for liquids for the return flight.

Avoid packing valuables such as a laptop, camera or personal digital assistants (PDAs), etc., in your suitcase in case of theft.

## Some ideas for your toiletries/liquids bag

- Pack any liquid medications you need for the flight in your carry-on bag. Pack them into your liquids bag if they will fit as this will make the security procedure smoother. Check your airport or airline website for advice.
- Even on a fairly short flight, taking a travel size toothbrush and toothpaste can be a good idea – their use can make you feel refreshed.
- For long flights, take small bottles of intensive moisturizing and hand lotions and a lip balm to hydrate skin.
- Aromatherapy products can help you to feel more relaxed. 'Roll on' products with essential oils such as lavender are the classic choice. Origins 'Peace of Mind' is based on peppermint oil and can help you to keep calm and alert.
- It is important to be hydrated and you may not be able to fit a bottle of water in your liquids bag. Make sure you have some spare change and buy a bottle once you are through security on your way to the lounge or departure gate.

## Checklist for an accompanying friend or relative

If there is someone travelling with you and it's appropriate to share information about your anxiety with them, they can be a very useful source of support. Many people will tend to deal with anxiety in others by offering reassurance and may not know how else to help. Reassurance is a bonus but may not be the most helpful way to assist you, as you now have many skills and techniques which are more appropriate to your own fear of flying. This checklist is designed for the use of your travelling companion, but it will help you both decide what type of support is most likely to help reduce your anxiety:

- Before you travel, try and make time to talk about how you can help. Ask the person you're flying with what happens when he or she becomes anxious – does he become silent or chatty? Does she 'freeze', withdraw or try and run away?
- What techniques has the person thought about using? It might help to know why he is taking this flight or if he has practised breathing or relaxation techniques.
- What is she going to use to distract herself (puzzles, music, reading material, etc.)?
- If you have time, read through the parts of this book that the person you are travelling with found most helpful, so that you can reinforce these with him or her as necessary.
- If you can, make sure the person you are accompanying has something to eat before travelling to the airport and gets a reasonable night's sleep before the flight. Plan your journey to the airport so that you have extra time to check in and get through security.
- Make sure that the person you are flying with has brought travel documents, snack food and whatever he or she plans to use to distract him or herself.
- If there is a long wait to board the flight and your companion is becoming anxious, try and give her something to do, even if it's only completing a crossword, counting the number of people wearing red or identifying as many airline logos as possible!
- During the flight, it can be very tempting to 'hover' and continually try to offer reassurance. This is very well intentioned and caring but it might not be the most helpful thing you can do. Try not to watch your travelling companion all the time but keep an eye out for symptoms of anxiety, especially those you have talked about before flying. If acceptable to both of you, hold his or her hand.
- If the person you are flying with does become anxious, remind him or her of the information and skills he or she decided to use from this book. A reminder that take-off is noisy but will not last very long may be helpful, for example, or you could suggest practising a breathing or relaxation technique as a means of distraction.
- Remember that you can ask for help from the cabin crew any time you need it. They are trained in how to deal with panic attacks and hyperventilation, so even if this does happen, they can assist you. Remember that a panic attack is frightening to encounter but

isn't necessarily damaging, and can go away quite quickly if treated appropriately.

## Using psychological skills and techniques

There is a lot of information in this book and you may not have time to read it all again just before you fly. This list gives you a summary of the techniques explained in the book so that you can remind yourself of the ones you have decided to try. Try not to constantly 'watch' yourself for signs of anxiety. Paying too much attention to the possibility that you might start to become anxious will actually help increase your anxiety. If you do notice that you are becoming anxious, here is a list of techniques we have covered in the book which should help:

- Plan ahead: what are the thoughts that you decided were most likely to make you anxious? How did you decide to change these so that they are more realistic and less likely to provoke anxiety? Remind yourself to notice these automatic thoughts and challenge them in the ways you have practised.
- What relaxation or breathing techniques have you decided to try? If you use music or recorded instructions to help you with these techniques, make sure you take them in your cabin bag.
- If you're travelling with someone who knows you may be anxious, have you used the checklist earlier in this chapter to let them know how best to help you?
- If you are becoming anxious, particularly if you notice some of the bodily sensations of anxiety, practise your breathing or relaxation techniques. If you cannot remember them, the simplest exercise is to breathe in for a count of five and then out for a count of five. You need to do this for at least a minute to start reducing anxiety.
- Be aware of any anxious or negative thoughts, and either challenge them in the way you have practised or use the thought-stopping techniques from Chapter 7.
- If they are thoughts you have not considered while working through this book, remember to look for thinking errors and correct them as you have practised.
- Make yourself as comfortable as possible: use blankets and pillows if they have been provided; remember the soothing items you have in your cabin bag and liquids bag.
- Distract yourself with whatever you have brought with you, or with a movie if there is one to watch.
- If you are travelling with someone, talk to them; if you have used

the 'companion' checklist with them, ask them to remind you what techniques you decided to use.

- If you are travelling alone, consider telling the crew that you are anxious and asking them to 'drop by' every so often just to let you know that the flight is continuing as normal.
- Look around at other passengers: this may seem perverse but every fourth or fifth passenger is apprehensive. You are not alone in your thoughts and worries.
- Remember that no flight lasts forever and that you have planned a reward.

Keep practising the techniques which work between flights and try not to leave a very long period of time before flying again.

## Turbulence

We have included a detailed list of techniques to use if you encounter turbulence because so many people tell us that they find it difficult to manage their anxiety about this. The following points will help if you become anxious about turbulence when flying:

- Turbulence may feel uncomfortable, but it cannot be considered a danger to the aircraft. Planes are built with turbulence in mind; they are hundreds of times stronger than the effects of bumpiness.
- Turbulence needs to be psychologically 'downgraded', from very threatening to something that is unwelcome but manageable.
- Many passengers dislike turbulence because they do not understand what is happening; it is simply air currents meeting the plane. Aircraft encounter this during every journey, although on some flights it may be more noticeable than on others. It is therefore a normal and expected part of air travel. On some journeys it will be more memorable, while on other occasions turbulence will not feature at all.
- Everyone on the plane is experiencing the same as what you are feeling; you are not alone in your feelings. However, different people think about what is happening differently. The pilots and crew have experienced this hundreds, if not thousands of times before. Your goal is to try to mimic what you think the crew will be feeling and experiencing. Ask yourself: 'How come they manage this all effortlessly while perhaps other passengers and I do not?' Think of at least three possible reasons. Can you now apply any of these insights into your own situation?

- Turbulence is limited in its duration. Say to yourself: 'My stress will come to an end; it always does. This "event" and experience of turbulence is but a blip in my life; it is really insignificant.'
- For some people, turbulence triggers two psychological reactions. First, it can switch on the mechanism that raises our anxiety levels. This is because the sensation of turbulence is unfamiliar and also unwelcome; we don't feel in control of it and we may associate it with unpleasant memories from another trip. Second, it leads to fatigue and stress because the balance centre in our ear is being over-stimulated.
- Say to yourself: 'I need to distract myself to reduce my anxiety and physical tension.' Watch the movie; start your relaxation techniques (breathing etc.); talk to the person next to you; read; listen to music or hum to yourself. It is always important to anticipate anxious and stressful times on your flight and your bag needs to be packed with things that can help to distract your thoughts. If you must, pass the time by counting the bumps and categorizing them into 1 (light), 2 (moderate) or 3 (very uncomfortable). Keep a running total – if there is no turbulence for three minutes, then you have to zero your score.
- Think differently about the effects of the motion: notice that some of us associate bumpiness and rocking with soothing moments in our lives. For example, think about what you are going through as being akin to sitting on a rocking chair and relaxing, or the soothing experience of being rocked in your pram or cradle as an infant. Developmentally, motion can be associated with soothing feelings, reassurance, safety and comfort, and we need to retrain ourselves to think of it differently. Your goal could be seen as to stop it automatically triggering what seems like a faulty fire alarm warning within yourself, or at least to ignore it once you have established that there is no real fire.

## When you return home

When you finish travelling, set aside a few minutes to think about what worked and whether you need to do anything differently next time:

- Make sure that you congratulate and reward yourself. Well done!
- What did you actually think when flying? Was it what you expected and were you able to use your new realistic interpretations of what was happening? Do you need to look at Chapters 6, 7, 8 or 9 again to remind yourself?

- Did the distractions you used work? If not, do you know why and can you think of any better ones for your next flight?
- Can you remember when you were most anxious or physically tense? What might help next time?
- Was there anything you wish you had taken with you that would have helped to reduce your anxiety even more? Make a note to take it with you next time.
- Where are you going to go next? Book another flight soon and continue to practise the techniques that have worked for you.

## Congratulations!

If you have worked with the techniques in this book and made progress in reducing your anxiety, well done! It takes hard work and commitment to overcome fears and anxiety and you should be proud of any progress you make. Overcoming your fear of flying is likely to be a slow and gradual change, as we said at the start of this book. As you start to overcome your fear of flying, continue to practise the techniques that work best for you and add others if you need to. Each step you take towards being able to fly with better managed anxiety, however small, is something we would like you to notice and be proud of. We hope you enjoy being able to travel to those places only sensibly accessible by flying – the world is there to explore!

If you have worked through this book and find that you have not made as much progress as you would like, it may be sensible to consider consulting a psychologist. This does not mean that you have failed to sort the problem out, or that you have deep problems. It simply means that, although this book will probably have helped you make some progress, it has not enabled you to completely overcome your fear. It may be that another factor or problem is driving your fear of flying. Working with a psychologist, as many of the case studies in Chapter 2 show, can be a rapid and effective way to make further progress towards overcoming your fear of flying. A psychologist can work with your unique fear in a way not completely possible here. There is a list of sources of further help to help you find a suitable psychologist after this chapter.

Overcoming a fear of flying is a challenge. Although this book provides a solid foundation in the skills and techniques that reduce anxiety associated with air travel, there are a number of reasons why a self-help book may not be the final step in becoming a confident flyer. First, there is not enough space in one book to cover every possible psychological technique that might help. Second, people differ a great deal in the way in which they learn to apply skills and techniques. Any book is limited in the extent to which it can assist you in using and developing these skills. Although this book reflects a great deal of the diversity we encounter in practice with fearful flyers, it cannot cover every way in which a fear of flying manifests. Nor can it completely take the place of a therapeutic conversation with a qualified psychologist. Sometimes, more than a self-help book will be needed.

By reading this book you will have learnt a considerable amount about modern psychological methods for treating anxiety and panic attacks. It may well be that you can apply some of these skills to similar problems in other areas of your life.

# Other sources of help

This is a list of other sources of help and information to assist you in overcoming your fear of flying.

## Books

The following books cover more of the technical aspects of flying than we have room for in this book. If you have read Chapters 7 and 9 and still need more information, one of these will probably have the answer:

John D. Anderson, *Introduction to Flight*. McGraw Hill International, 2008.

Written for undergraduate engineers, so it is fairly technical, but it will answer almost any technical questions about aircraft and flight.

Trevor Thom, *The Air Pilot's Manual, Vol 4: The Aeroplane Technical*. Airlife Publishing, 2003.

This is the book student pilots use to prepare for their first licence. It has many clear explanations and diagrams and should answer most questions.

## Psychologists

If you want to work with a psychologist to make more progress on overcoming your fear of flying, contact us. Our website is <www. FearOfFlyingExperts.com>. You can also find local psychologists on the British Psychological Society's website <www.bps.org.uk>

## One further useful contact:

Virtual Aviation provide simulator experiences specifically designed to help overcome a fear of flying. If you think this might be a useful part of your graded practice as described in Chapter 7, their website is <www.virtualaviation.co.uk>.

# Index